W9-APC-996

Acute Care Nurse Practitioner Certification Study Question Book

EDITOR

**Sally K. Miller, M.S., R.N.,C.S., C.R.N.P.,
C.C.R.N., A.N.P., G.N.P., A.C.N.P.**
Vice-President
Health Leadership Associates, Inc.
Potomac, Maryland

Adjunct Lecturer
College of Nursing
Rutgers, the State University of New Jersey
Newark, New Jersey

Clinical Assistant Professor
School of Nursing
University of Medicine and Dentistry of New Jersey
Newark, New Jersey

Health Leadership Associates
Potomac, Maryland

Question Books

Family Nurse Practitioner Certification Study Question Set

(ISBN 1-878028-26-X)

by
Health Leadership Associates, Inc.

Consists of
The

**Adult Nurse Practitioner Certification
Study Question Book
ISBN 1-878028-20-0**

**Pediatric Nurse Practitioner Certification
Study Question Book
ISBN 1-878028-21-9**

**Women's Health Nurse Practitioner
Certification Study Question Book
ISBN 1-878028-22-7**

Additional Nursing Certification Study Question Books by Health Leadership Associates, Inc.

Acute Care Nurse Practitioner Certification Study Question Book
(ISBN# 1-878028-25-1), List Price $30.00

Adult Nurse Practitioner Certification Study Question Book
(ISBN# 1-878028-20-0), List Price $30.00

Pediatric Nurse Practitioner Certification Study Question Book
(ISBN# 1-878028-21-9), List Price $30.00

Women's Health Care Nurse Practitioner Certification Study Question Book
(ISBN# 1-878028-22-7), List Price $30.00

Family Nurse Practitioner Certification Study Question Book Set
(This shrink wrapped set consists of the Adult, Pediatric, and Women's Health Study Question Books).
(ISBN# 1-878028-26-X). List Price $60.00

Certification Review Books

Family Nurse Practitioner Set

(ISBN 1-878028-24-3)

by
Health Leadership Associates, Inc.

Consists of
The

**Adult Nurse Practitioner Certification
Review Guide
(3rd edition)**

**Pediatric Nurse Practitioner Certification
Review Guide
(3rd edition)**

**Women's Health Care Nurse Practitioner
Certification Review Guide**

Health Leadership Associates, Inc.
Managing Editor: Virginia Layng Millonig
                     Mary A. Millonig
Production Manager: Martha M. Pounsberry
Editorial Assistants: Bridget M. Jones
                       Cheryl C. Patterson
Cover and Design: Merrifield Graphics
Composition: Port City Press, Inc.
Design and Production: Port City Press, Inc.

Printed in the United States of America

Health Leadership Associates, Inc.
P.O. Box 59153
Potomac, Maryland 20859

Library of Congress Cataloging-in-Publication Data

Acute care nurse practitioner certification study question book
    Sally K. Miller, contributing authors,
    Lynn Kelso ... [et al.].
      Includes bibliographical references
      ISBN 1-878028-25-1
        1. Nurse practitioners—Examinations, questions, etc.   2. Primary nursing—Examinations,
questions, etc.   I. Miller, Sally K.
II. Lynn Kelso
    [DNLM: 1. Nurse Practitioner certification examination study questions.   2. Nursing
Care examination questions.
10 9 8 7 6 5 4 3 2 1

NOTICE: The editors, authors and publisher of this book have taken care that the information and recommendations contained herein are accurate and compatible with standards generally accepted at the time of publication. However, the editors, authors and publisher cannot accept responsibility for errors or omissions or for the consequences from application of the information in this book and make no warranty, express or implied with respect to the contents of the book.

Contributing Authors

Lynn A. Kelso, M.S.N., R.N.,C.S., A.C.N.P., C.C.R.N.
Assistant Professor
College of Nursing
University of Kentucky
Pulmonary/Critical Care Department
A. B. Chandler Medical Center
Lexington, Kentucky

Ruth M. Kleinpell, Ph.D., R.N.,C.S., A.C.N.P., C.C.R.N.
Associate Professor
Department of Medical-Surgical Nursing
College of Nursing
Rush University
Chicago, Illinois

Candis Morrison, Ph.D., R.N.,C.S., A.C.N.P.
Assistant Professor
School of Nursing
Johns Hopkins University
Baltimore, Maryland

Reviewers

Mary E. Elmer, M.S.N., R.N.,C.S., C.R.N.P., A.C.N.P.
Associate Medical Program Coordinator
Clinical Research
Merck Research Laboratories
Merck & Co., Inc.
West Point, Pennsylvania

Marguerite Lovett Knox, M.N., R.N.,C.S., A.N.P. A.C.N.P., C.C.R.N.
Clinical Assistant Professor
College of Nursing
University of South Carolina
Columbia, South Carolina

Sally K. Miller, M.S., R.N.,C.S., C.R.N.P., C.C.R.N., A.N.P., G.N.P., A.C.N.P.
Vice-President
Health Leadership Associates, Inc.
Potomac, Maryland
Adjunct Lecturer
College of Nursing
Rutgers, the State University of New Jersey
Newark, New Jersey
Clinical Assistant Professor
School of Nursing
University of Medicine and Dentistry of New Jersey
Newark, New Jersey

Preface

Health Leadership Associates is pleased to introduce one more component to our complement of Nurse Practitioner Certification Review materials. This "Acute Care Nurse Practitioner Certification Study Question Book" will further assist the user of this book to be successful in the examination process. It should by no means be the only source used for preparation for the Acute Care Nurse Practitioner Certification examination. It has been developed primarily to enhance your test taking skills while also integrating the principles (becoming test-wise) of test taking found in the "Test Taking Strategies and Skills" chapter of the "Adult Nurse Practitioner Certification Review Guide" published by Health Leadership Associates. Content for the examination, based upon the content outline from the ANCC, can be found in the "Acute Care Nurse Practitioner Certification Review Course." Together the course and/or home study program provide a comprehensive and total approach to success in the examination process. They enable the users of these materials to be successful in the test taking process, and reinforce the knowledge base that is critical in the delivery of care in the practice setting. Many individuals feel that taking practice test questions is the most important factor in the certification examination preparation process, yet it is but one strategy to be used in combination with a strong knowledge base. Success in the certification examination area is based upon both excellent test taking skills and a comprehensive understanding of the content of the examination. As a nurse practitioner seeking certification, it is important to not lose sight of the definition and purpose of certification. "Certification is a process by which nongovernmental agencies or associations confirm that an individual licensed to practice as a professional has met certain predetermined standards specified by that profession for specialty practice." Its purpose is to assure the public that an individual has mastered a body of knowledge and acquired skills in a particular specialty (ANA, 1979).

Inherent to the preparation for certification examinations is rigorous attention to the directives and materials from the certification boards. Content outlines and sample test questions are often provided to examinees prior to the examinations. Specifics for each examination including suggested readings will be provided by the individual testing boards.

This question book has been prepared by board certified nurse practitioners. The questions have then been reviewed and critiqued by board certified nurse practitioners (content experts) and a test construction specialist. There are 300 problem oriented certification board-type multiple choice questions which are divided according to content area (based upon testing board content outlines) with answers, rationales and a reference list. Every effort has been made to develop sample questions that are representative of the types of questions that may be found on the certification examinations, however, style and format of the examination may differ. Engaging in the exercise of test taking, an understanding of test taking strategies and, knowledge in respective content areas can only lead to success.

CONTENTS

Health Promotion and Risk Assessment for Age Cohort

Lynn A. Kelso

Select one best answer to the following questions.

1. A 53-year-old male is ready for discharge after a three-vessel coronary artery bypass graft (CABG). He has a 43-pack-year history of smoking and has discussed his desire to stop smoking. While implementing patient teaching the acute care nurse practitioner (ACNP) tells the patient that:

   a. Elimination of cigarettes from the house is essential
   b. He will experience withdrawal after three days
   c. He may feel tired and nauseated
   d. He needs to seek counseling to quit

2. A 63-year-old female has been on estrogen replacement therapy since undergoing a total abdominal hysterectomy eight years ago. She has a family history of osteoporosis and asks about preventive measures. The ACNP should tell her that:

   a. She should take 500 mg of calcium per day
   b. Walking will help protect bone mass
   c. She may take calcitonin three times per week
   d. She should be evaluated more often because of her family history

3. A 41-year-old married female is admitted via the emergency department with multiple fractures after a motor vehicle accident. Upon further assessment three large ecchymotic areas are noted on her upper thighs, and radiology reports three healed fractures visible in her upper extremities. The ACNP should:

   a. Report findings to the local authorities
   b. Discuss the case with a social worker
   c. Provide her with information about shelters
   d. Question her about her history with violence

4. The ACNP is discussing exercise with a 49-year-old male who is concerned about his health status. He states that he is trying to go to the gym three times a week. The ACNP explains that:

   a. Achieving maximal heart rate for 20 minutes, three times a week, is adequate
   b. After the age of 50 exercise does not decrease the risk of heart disease
   c. Moderate activity for 30 minutes most or all days of the week is preferable
   d. Any exercise that he undertakes will decrease the risk of heart disease

5. While speaking at a patient program for health promotion, you inform patients that the most effective way to improve health and to decrease the risk of cancer is to:

   a. Increase physical activity
   b. Use a sunscreen
   c. Stop smoking
   d. Decrease fat intake

6. You are doing a health evaluation of a 42-year-old female. She has annual gynecological evaluations, and routine dental and eye care. She has no medical problems and a benign family history. She has no record of blood work screening. Based upon current guidelines for health screening you suggest that the patient:

   a. Have a cholesterol level drawn
   b. Continue her current routine
   c. Schedule a baseline electrocardiogram (ECG)
   d. Should have liver function tests (LFT)

7. A 64-year-old Korean female is being evaluated for lower back pain. Her past medical history is unremarkable except for premature menopause at age 48. She is on no medication and she has a 24 pack year smoking history. Your initial orders should include:

   a. Serum calcium and phosphorus
   b. Bone densitometry
   c. Serum alkaline phosphatase
   d. Magnetic resonance imaging (MRI) of the spine

8. A 57-year-old black male is being assessed preoperatively. He complains of hip pain, urinary frequency and awakening at night to void. His past medical

history is unremarkable. He does not smoke or drink. The ACNP should consider ordering:

    a. A prostate specific antigen (PSA) level
    b. A glucose tolerance test (GTT)
    c. A urology consult
    d. A hip radiograph

9. The ACNP is evaluating a 35-year-old female. She is six weeks postpartum with her first child. Her past medical history (PMH) is unremarkable and her family history includes a maternal grandmother with breast cancer. The patient should be encouraged to:

    a. Have a mammogram
    b. Have a breast ultrasound
    c. Do regular self-breast examinations
    d. Only breast feed for three months

10. A 21-year-old female presents for a routine physical examination. She complains of fatigue and diarrhea, but has gained four pounds in three weeks. Her physical examination is unremarkable except for bruising of three fingers on her right hand and excoriation of her pharynx. Based upon these assessment findings the ACNP should focus the history on:

    a. Feelings of depression
    b. Date of last menstrual period
    c. History of weight loss/gain
    d. Illicit drug use

11. A 42-year-old African-American female is seen for a routine physical examination. During the examination she has no complaints and her history is benign. For screening purposes the ACNP should order a:

    a. Total cholesterol
    b. Glaucoma screening
    c. Sigmoidoscopy
    d. Colonoscopy

12. A 21-year-old white male is admitted for a herniorrhaphy. Because you are aware of the leading causes of mortality for this age cohort, the history should include asking this patient about:

    a. Self-testicular examination
    b. Helmet use while biking

    c. Seat belt use

    d. Alcohol intake

13. A Native-American male, age 42, is being re-evaluated for hypertension. The ACNP should order additional laboratory tests including:

    a. Total bilirubin

    b. Fasting blood glucose

    c. PSA

    d. Creatine kinase (CK) and isoenzymes

14. A 54-year-old male is hospitalized following a motor vehicle accident (MVA). He has no significant medical history. You recommend that he see his primary care physician following discharge for routine evaluation which should include a(n):

    a. Upper endoscopy

    b. Sigmoidoscopy

    c. Colonoscopy

    d. Barium swallow

15. You are evaluating a 78-year-old male in the emergency department for altered level of consciousness. His daughter says that although he was fine the day before, this is just normal aging and she would like to take him home. The appropriate action for the ACNP would be to:

    a. Discharge the patient to home

    b. Recommend nursing home placement

    c. Admit for a full diagnostic evaluation

    d. Evaluate for elder abuse

Answers and Rationale

1. **(c)** The most common manifestations of withdrawal from nicotine include drowsiness, headache, increased appetite, sleep disturbances, and gastrointestinal (GI) complaints. These symptoms will usually begin within 24 hours of smoking cessation. Since it is stated in the stem that the patient has discussed his desire to stop smoking, it is now important that he be made aware of withdrawal symptoms so that he may cope with them effectively (Larson, p. 73).

2. **(b)** Weight bearing exercise for one hour, three times a week, helps to protect bone mass. Recommended calcium intake is 1500 mg/day. Calcitonin may be used to treat established osteoporosis (Dagogo-Jack, p. 453).

3. **(d)** When assessing for domestic violence, questions should focus on establishing a history of violence. You do not have a case to report to authorities, and although discussing the case with a social worker may help you in determining your actions, the best way to begin helping the patient is to establish that there is a history of domestic violence (Komaroff, p. 23).

4. **(c)** The NIH Consensus Development Conference on Physical Activity and Cardiovascular Health states that a goal for exercise should be to accumulate at least 30 minutes of moderate intensity physical activity on most, or all, days of the week (Jones, p. 88).

5. **(c)** The #1 cancer prevention, for many types of cancer, is to stop smoking. Using sunscreen will help to prevent skin cancer, and increased activity does help to decrease the risk of breast and colon cancer (McPhee, p. 5).

6. **(b)** The American College of Physicians no longer recommends serum cholesterol levels for males under the age of 35 or females under the age of 45 unless there is a family history of lipoprotein disorder, or the patient has two risk factors for coronary artery disease (Connelly, p. 48).

7. **(b)** Risk factors for the development of osteoporosis include females of Caucasian or Asian descent, early menopause, and therapy with glucocorticoids. Bone mass measurements are sensitive and specific for osteopenia and predict the risk of fractures. Serum calcium and phosphorus levels are normal

with osteoporosis and alkaline phosphatase levels may only be elevated after a fracture (Dagogo-Jack, p. 450).

8. **(c)** African-American males have the highest incidence of prostate cancer in the world. Common complaints of advanced stages of prostate cancer include back and hip pain, bladder pain, and perineal or rectal pain. PSA levels are useful to assess for recurrence, for bulk of disease, and may be helpful to detect prostate cancer in asymptomatic patients. With this patient's presentation it is most important that he be seen by a urologist and continue his evaluation for prostate cancer (Vetrosky, p. 90).

9. **(a)** Women who have their first term pregnancy after the age of 30 have an increased risk of breast cancer. This risk increases if the first term pregnancy is after the age of 35. A baseline mammogram should be done and is recommended between the ages of 35 to 40 (White, p. 83).

10. **(a)** Bulimia is a greater risk in young adult women. Patients suffering from bulimia frequently complain of bloating, fatigue and diarrhea. Weight either does not change or there may be an increase in weight. The bruising of the fingers is commonly seen in bulimia secondary to inducing vomiting, which causes the excoriation of the pharynx. Depression and feelings of inadequacy or loss of control are frequently associated with bulimia (Grinenko, p. 699).

11. **(b)** It is recommended that African-American women be screened for glaucoma after the age of 40. Caucasian women should be screened after the age of 50. Sigmoidoscopy is not recommended for screening until after age 50, and stool for occult blood is not specific (Komaroff, p. 22).

12. **(c)** The leading cause of death in white males under the age of 24 is MVA, with young adult drivers having the highest rate of motor vehicle fatalities. Young African-American males are seven times more likely to die secondary to homicide than Caucasian or Asian males (Irwin, p. 33).

13. **(b)** The American Diabetes Association (ADA) recommends fasting blood glucose screening every three years after the age of 45, or younger in persons at risk for developing diabetes mellitus. Risk factors include obesity, race/ethnicity (African-American, Native American, Hispanic, Asian-Americans,

and Pacific-Islanders), age over 45, and hypertension (Report of the Expert Committee on the Diagnosis and Classification of Diabetes Mellitus, p. S-15).

14. **(b)** Both the American Cancer Society and the U.S. Preventive Services Task Force recommend a screening sigmoidoscopy after the age of 50. These groups have not yet made recommendations for how often a sigmoidoscopy should be done. Colonoscopy is cumbersome and too invasive for widespread screening (Brawley, p. 504).

15. **(c)** An abrupt decline in any system or function is always due to some disease. It can not be attributed to normal aging (Resnick, p. 37).

References

Brawley, O. W., & Kramer, B. S. (1998). Prevention and early detection of cancer. In A. S. Fauci, E. Braunwald, K. J. Isselbacher, J. D. Wilson, J. B. Martin, D. L. Kasper, S. L. Hauser, & D. L. Longo (Eds.), *Harrison's principles of internal medicine* (14th ed., pp. 499-505). NY: McGraw-Hill.

Connelly, M. T., & Inui, T. S. (1998). Principles of disease prevention. In A. S. Fauci, E. Braunwald, K. J. Isselbacher, J. D. Wilson, J. B. Martin, D. L. Kasper, S. L. Hauser, & D. L. Longo (Eds.), *Harrison's principles of internal medicine* (14th ed., pp. 46-48). NY: McGraw-Hill.

Dagogo-Jack, S. (1998). Mineral and metabolic bone diseases. In C. F. Carey, H. H. Lee, & K. F. Woeltje (Eds.), *The Washington manual of medical therapeutics* (29th ed., pp. 441-455). Philadelphia: Lippincott-Raven.

Grinenko, D. M. (1996). Anorexia and bulimia nervosa. In R. E. Rakel, & R. M. Kleberg (Eds.), *Saunders manual of medical practice.* (pp. 699-701). Philadelphia: W. B. Saunders.

Irwin, C. E., & Shafer, M. A. (1998). Adolescent health problems. In A. S. Fauci, E. Braunwald, K. J. Isselbacher, J. D. Wilson, J. B. Martin, D. L. Kasper, S. L. Hauser, & D. L. Longo (Eds.), *Harrison's principles of internal medicine* (14th ed., pp. 30-37). NY: McGraw-Hill.

Jones, K. D., & Jones, J. M. (1997). Physical exercise. *Clinician Reviews, 7*(3), 81-104.

Komaroff, A. L., Robb-Nicholson, C., & Woo, B. (1998). Women's health. In A. S. Fauci, E. Braunwald, K. J. Isselbacher, J. D. Wilson, J. B. Martin, D. L. Kasper, S. L. Hauser, & D. L. Longo (Eds.), *Harrison's principles of internal medicine* (14th ed., pp. 21-24). NY: McGraw-Hill.

Larson, D. (1997). Smoking cessation: Counseling your patients. *Clinician Reviews, 7*(6), 57-80.

McPhee, S. J. & Schroeder, S. A. (1998). General approach to the patient: Health maintenance and disease prevention and common symptoms. In L. M. Tierney, Jr., S. J. McPhee, & M. A. Papadakis (Eds.), *Current medical diagnosis and treatment* (37th ed., pp. 1-29). Stamford, CT: Appleton & Lange.

Report of the expert committee on the diagnosis and classification of diabetes mellitus. (1998). *Diabetes Care, 21* (Supplement 1), S5-S19.

Resnick, N. M. (1998). Geriatric medicine. In A. S. Fauci, E. Braunwald, K. J. Isselbacher, J. D. Wilson, J. B. Martin, D. L. Kasper, S. L. Hauser, & D. L. Longo

(Eds.), *Harrison's principles of internal medicine* (14th ed., pp. 37-46). NY: McGraw-Hill.

Vetrosky, D. T., Gerdom, L., & White, G. L. (1997). Prostate cancer: Pathology, diagnosis, and management. *Clinician Reviews, 7*(5), 79-100.

White, G. L., & Griffith, C. J. (1996). Breast cancer: Reducing mortality through early detection. *Clinician Reviews, 6*(9), 79-83.

Risk Factor Considerations and Prevention

Lynn A. Kelso

Select one best answer to the following questions.

1. A 30-year-old female with a family history of breast cancer presents for a physical examination. When discussing additional risk factors you ask about:

    a. How many sexual partners she has had
    b. Fluctuations in her weight
    c. Age at menarche
    d. Any previous abortions

2. You are assessing a 23-year-old male who works as a lifeguard. He has three nevi on his upper back. They are all symmetrical and dark brown and range in size from 3 mm to 6.3 mm. The next appropriate step would be to:

    a. Question about family history
    b. Teach skin self evaluation
    c. Encourage him to change professions
    d. Schedule for excision of nevi

3. A 45-year-old male is scheduled for a cholecystectomy. He has a history of gall stones and multiple bouts of cholangitis with partial and complete bile duct obstruction. During his preoperative assessment he complains of increased bruising and bleeding gums. Your preoperative orders include:

    a. Vitamin K 10 mEq SQ
    b. Platelets one 6 pack IV
    c. Desmopressin 25 μg IV
    d. Fresh frozen plasma (FFP) 4 units IV

4. You are performing a preoperative evaluation on a 51-year-old female scheduled for an elective knee replacement. Her past medical history is significant

for hypertension, diabetes mellitus (DM), and a myocardial infarction (MI) four months ago. The next appropriate step would be to:

    a. Schedule an ECG and echocardiogram
    b. Order a cardiology consult
    c. Postpone surgery for two months
    d. Proceed with your evaluation

5. A 30-year-old female has been in the emergency department three times for fractures which are a result of domestic violence. While discussing her options the ACNP attempts to establish her risk for increased violence by asking about:

    a. Access to firearms
    b. Marital counseling
    c. History of child abuse
    d. Her husband's occupation

6. A 26-year-old firefighter is being evaluated in the emergency department following severe smoke inhalation. During your assessment you notice 2nd degree burns on his neck and upper chest. He is complaining of dyspnea on exertion and lightheadedness. The most appropriate course of action would be to:

    a. Observe for four hours and then discharge
    b. Admit to the floor and observe for 24 hours
    c. Transfer to a burn unit for observation
    d. Admit to the intensive care unit (ICU) and consider intubation

7. A 47-year-old house painter is admitted via the emergency department with a three day history of nausea and vomiting accompanied by jaundice. His liver function studies are elevated. He is on no medications and does not smoke. He denies chronic alcohol ingestion and illicit drug use. When working up his liver abnormalities, the ACNP should consider:

    a. Work/chemical exposures
    b. A urine drug screen
    c. Past abdominal surgeries
    d. Risk factors for substance abuse

8. A 62-year-old female presents for a routine physical examination. Her personal and family history is unremarkable for heart disease except for a 36 pack year tobacco history, however she states that she stopped smoking at age 48. She asks about her risk for heart disease and you explain that:

    a. Smoking always increases the risk for ischemic heart disease

    b. Once you stop smoking your risk is cut in half

    c. After 10 to 14 years of not smoking there is no increased risk

    d. Risk factors, other than smoking, play a greater role in heart disease

9. A 31-year-old trauma victim required a splenectomy due to abdominal injuries. Upon recovery, your orders should include:

    a. Pneumococcal vaccine

    b. Influenza vaccine

    c. Granulocyte colony stimulating factor

    d. Hepatitis B immunoglobulin

10. You are immunizing the family of a patient who has hepatitis B. They have received their first dose and you tell them they must return to the clinic in:

    a. 1 month

    b. 1 and 6 months

    c. 1, 2, and 6 months

    d. 6 months

11. A 19-year-old female with human immunodeficiency virus (HIV) is being discharged after a herniorrhaphy. She has a history of asthma and is allergic to sulfa drugs. Her discharge medications should include:

    a. Pentamidine 300 mg inhaled once weekly

    b. Dapsone 100 mg p.o. q.d.

    c. Trimethoprim/sulfamethoxazole one tablet DS p.o. q.d.

    d. Clindamycin 600 mg p.o. b.i.d.

12. A 67-year-old female has a history of hypertension, chronic obstructive pulmonary disease (COPD), and Guillain-Barré syndrome. She is allergic to penicillin (PCN) and eggs. She has questions about receiving an influenza vaccine and the ACNP explains that:

    a. An allergy to PCN is a contraindication

    b. Patients with hypertension are at increased risk for influenza

    c. An allergy to eggs is a contraindication

    d. Influenza vaccines have no clear association with Guillain-Barré

13. When discussing the prevention of infectious diseases with a 21-year-old patient, the ACNP explains that the best way to prevent the biggest infectious disease threat in this age group is to:

    a. Have antibody titres and boosters if necessary

   b. Follow immunization recommendations
   c. Have an annual TB skin test
   d. Use condoms during sexual encounters

14. A 46-year-old male has been treated with a full course of chemotherapy. He is now being admitted with an altered mental status. His absolute neutrophil count is 284 cells/μL. To best prevent infection in this patient, initial orders should include:

   a. Strict handwashing
   b. Strict isolation
   c. Empiric antibiotics
   d. Granulocyte colony stimulating factor

Answers and Rationale

1. **(c)** Early menarche and late menopause are both considered risk factors for the development of breast cancer (White, p. 83).

2. **(a)** The warning signs for atypical mole syndrome include asymmetry, border irregularity, color variability, and diameter > 6 mm. With atypical mole syndrome, the greatest risk of developing malignant melanoma appears to be strongly dependent upon personal or family history of malignant melanoma. With a nevi that is > 8 mm in diameter, there is a greater risk for malignant melanoma and it should be excised and biopsied to rule out abnormal or malignant cells, however, any lesion that is suspected to be melanoma should be excised (McEldowney, p. 68).

3. **(a)** This patient is exhibiting signs of increased bleeding. Because of his history of bile duct obstruction, he may be unable to absorb Vitamin K secondary to loss of bile drainage. There is no history of liver dysfunction so administering Vitamin K should correct any coagulopathy (Galarraga, p. 23).

4. **(c)** A history of an MI within the past six months is a major risk factor for perioperative complications, including acute MI and sudden cardiac death. Elective surgery should be postponed until the patient is at least six months post MI (Galarraga, p. 22).

5. **(a)** When assessing the risk factors for escalating violence, there is an increased risk of injury or death in households where there is easy access to a firearm (Komaroff, p. 23).

6. **(d)** Because burns are located on the patient's chest and neck, there is a risk that he has burn injuries to his trachea. This could rapidly lead to a loss of airway and the need for intubation. This patient should be admitted to the ICU, closely monitored, and placed on humidified oxygen or be electively intubated in order to protect and maintain his airway (Goodenberger, p. 526).

7. **(a)** There are many hepatotoxic agents which may be found in the work place. These include carbon tetrachloride, found in solvents and cleaning fluids,

and metals, particularly arsenic, used in pesticides and paints. Using these paints in a poorly ventilated area can lead to hepatotoxicity (Hu, p. 20).

8. **(c)** The Nurses' Health Study has shown that when a woman stops smoking, $\frac{1}{3}$ of her risk for ischemic heart disease is eliminated within two years, and any additional risk was eliminated 10 to 14 years after smoking cessation. Although family history plays a significant role in the development of heart disease, this patient's family history is negative, and so smoking is her only potential risk factor (Komaroff, p. 22).

9. **(a)** Patients are at risk for developing pneumococcal pneumonia after a splenectomy. These patients should receive a pneumococcal vaccine to prevent this (Fraser, p. 556).

10. **(b)** Recombinant HbsAg is given in a series of three injections at 0, 1, and 6 months (Fraser, p. 556).

11. **(b)** HIV positive patients with CD4$^+$ counts less than 200 cells/μL should receive prophylaxis for PCP. Prophylaxis can be accomplished with trimethoprim/sulfamethoxazol (TMP/SMX), pentamidine, or dapsone. Her sulfa allergy prevents her from taking TMP/SMX and she may not tolerate inhaled pentamidine because of her asthma. Dapsone would be the prophylaxis of choice in this patient (Tebas, p. 294).

12. **(c)** Yearly influenza vaccines should be given to patients over the age of 65. There is no contraindication for hypertension or for a PCN allergy, however, an allergy to chicken eggs, or any other components of the vaccine, is a contraindication (Shandera, p. 1256).

13. **(d)** The major infectious disease problem in the Western world is AIDS. Using condoms and practicing safe sex techniques has been demonstrated to decrease the risk of HIV transmission (McPhee, p. 4).

14. **(a)** In preventing infection in neutropenic patients, nothing has proven to be more effective than strict handwashing techniques. Although GCSF may be ordered, it is extremely expensive and you should know the trend in the patient's absolute neurtophil count (Tebas, p. 298).

References

Fraser, V. J., & Woeltje, K. F. (1998). Immunizations and postexposure therapies. In C. F. Carey, H. H. Lee, & K. F. Woeltje (Eds.), *The Washington manual of medical therapeutics* (29th ed., pp. 556-559). Philadelphia: Lippincott-Raven.

Galarraga, J. (1996). Preoperative evaluation. In R. E. Rakel, & R. M. Kleberg (Eds.), *Saunders manual of medical practice* (pp. 22-25). Philadelphia: W. B. Saunders.

Goodenberg, D. (1998). Medical emergencies. In L. M. Tierney, Jr., S. J. McPhee, & M. A. Papadakis (Eds.), *Current medical diagnosis and treatment* (37th ed., pp. 494-526). Stamford, CT: Appleton & Lange.

Hu, H., & Speizer, F. E. (1998). Influence of environment and occupational hazards of disease. In A. S. Fauci, E. Braunwald, K. J. Isselbacher, J. D. Wilson, J. B. Martin, D. L. Kasper, S. L. Hauser, & D. L. Longo (Eds.), *Harrison's principles of internal medicine* (14th ed., pp. 18-21). NY: McGraw-Hill.

Komaroff, A. L., Robb-Nicholson, C., & Woo, B. (1998). Women's health. In A. S. Fauci, E. Braunwald, K. J. Isselbacher, J. D. Wilson, J. B. Martin, D. L. Kasper, S. L. Hauser, & D. L. Longo (Eds.), *Harrison's principles of internal medicine* (14th ed., pp. 21-24). NY: McGraw-Hill.

McEldowney, S. (1997). Malignant melanoma: Familial, genetic, and psychosocial factors. *Clinician Reviews, 7*(7), 65-82.

McPhee, S. J., & Schroeder, S. A. (1998). General approach to the patient: Health maintenance and disease prevention and common symptoms. In L. M. Tierney, Jr., S. J. McPhee, & M. A. Papadakis (Eds.), *Current medical diagnosis and treatment* (37th ed., pp. 1-29). Stamford, CT: Appleton & Lange.

Shandera, W. X., & Carlini, M. E. (1998). Infectious disease: Viral and rickettsial. In L. M. Tierney, Jr., S. J. McPhee, & M. A. Papadakis (Eds.), *Current medical diagnosis and treatment* (37th ed., pp. 1231-1266). Stamford, CT: Appleton & Lange.

Tebas, P., & Horgan, M. (1998). The immunocompromised host. In C. F. Carey, H. H. Lee, & K. F. Woeltje (Eds.), *The Washington manual of medical therapeutics* (29th ed., pp. 288-301). Philadelphia: Lippincott-Raven.

White, G. L., & Griffith, C. J. (1996). Breast cancer: reducing mortality through early detection. *Clinician Reviews, 6*(9), 77-106.

Dermatological Disorders

Candis Morrison

Select one best answer to the following questions.

1. A 22-year-old presents with a history of intermittent episodes of red patches on his knees, elbows, and posterior scalp. These are well demarcated and are covered with silvery scales. There is minimal to no itching. He has attempted self treatment with calamine lotion and antihistamine cream. There are no systemic signs or symptoms. Which of the following conditions is the most likely etiology?

    a. Candidiasis
    b. Seborrheic dermatitis
    c. Tinea corporis
    d. Psoriasis

2. An otherwise healthy patient develops a new rash. He describes it as mildly pruritic. On examination the lesions are oval, fawn colored, and appear to follow lines of cleavage on the trunk. You suspect pityriasis rosea. Which test is indicated in this situation?

    a. Rapid plasma reagin
    b. Throat culture
    c. Lyme titer
    d. Antinuclear antibodies

Questions 3 and 4 refer to the following scenario.

As the ACNP you are caring for a 24-year-old woman with a history of recurrent urinary tract infections. She was started on prophylactic sulfonamides two weeks ago. On day 10 of therapy she became slightly febrile and very fatigued. She then developed circular erythematous lesions from 0.5 cm to 3 cm in size all over her body. Some blistered lesions were evident. The lesions are flat, have pale centers, and are present on her palms and soles. They are nonpruritic. She also developed oral muco-sal lesions which now appear as shallow ulcers, and she is having severe dysuria.

3. This clinical picture is consistent with which of the following diagnoses?

    a. Urticaria
    b. Pemphigus vulgaris
    c. Primary syphilis
    d. Stevens-Johnson syndrome

4. Treatment of this patient involves:

    a. Supportive care
    b. Antihistamines
    c. IV antibiotics
    d. Topical steroids

5. R. K. is a 33-year-old male with HIV. He complains of a three day history of severe, right sided, lower thoracic pain. Yesterday he began to develop small blisters on the skin over the painful area. On examination, you see grouped, deep seated vesicles on the posterior trunk at the level of the tenth thoracic ver-tebra. They stop at the midline. Treatment for this symptom complex should in-clude:

    a. Acyclovir 800 mg, five times per day for at least seven days
    b. Cephalexin 50 mg/kg/day for 10 days
    c. 1% cortisone ointment b.i.d. p.r.n.
    d. Griseofulvin 30mg/kg/day for one week

6. A 22-year-old is seen for an ''infected face.'' Three days ago she noted increas-ing redness around a small pimple on her forehead. It became tender and slightly warm. Today she noted expanding redness and more pain. On examina-tion her temperature is 38.2° C. In the right frontal area there is a 3 mm pus-tule with 4 cm of surrounding induration. It encompasses the eyebrow and up-per lid margin. The entire area is warm to touch and tender to palpation. Immediate treatment should include:

    a. Systemic steroids
    b. Incision and drainage
    c. Systemic antibiotics
    d. Topical antibiotics

Answers and Rationale

1. **(d)** The combination of red plaques and silvery scales on the elbows and knees with scaliness in the scalp is diagnostic of psoriasis. Skin biopsy would provide definitive diagnosis (Berger, p. 123).

2. **(a)** Though this rash is consistent with pityriasis rosea, a serologic test for syphilis should be performed. Secondary syphilis can present with any type of rash. It may be otherwise asymptomatic at this stage and is readily curable if detected. Pityriasis rosea is self limiting (Berger, p. 125).

3. **(d)** Erythema multiforme is divided into minor and major categories, dependent on the degree of mucosal involvement. Erythema multiforme major (Stevens-Johnson syndrome) is defined by systemic toxicity and involvement of two mucosal surfaces (in this case, oral and urethral). It is often associated with drugs; especially sulfonamides, NSAID, and anticonvulsants. Urticaria should be pruritic (Berger, pp. 151-152).

4. **(a)** The treatment of Stevens-Johnson syndrome is primarily supportive. Corticorsteroid use is controversial, however this would involve systemic administration. These patients require control of pain and surveillance for secondary infection. Patients with large areas of denuded skin need fluid and electrolyte management (Shaw & Robertson, p. 361).

5. **(a)** This scenario describes a typical case of herpes zoster. Pain follows the course of a nerve and is usually followed in about 48 hours by painful, grouped vesicular lesions. Involvement is unilateral and lesions are usually on the face or trunk. In immunocompromised patients, generalized life threatening dissemination may occur. High dose oral acyclovir should be initiated as soon as possible. Progression may necessitate IV acyclovir (Berger, pp. 137-138).

6. **(c)** Facial cellulitis is often treated with intravenous antibiotics because of the risk of cavernous sinus thrombosis. The usual treatment is a cephalosporin, a penicillinase-resistant penicillin, or clindamycin (Griffin, pp. 557, 622).

References

Bartlett, J. G. (1996). Infections of the skin, soft tissue and bone. In J. D. Stobo, D. B. Hellmann, P. W. Ladenson, B. G. Petty, & T. A. Traill (Eds.), *The principles and practice of medicine* (23rd ed.). Stamford, CT: Appleton & Lange.

Berger, T. G. (1998). Skin & appendages. In L. M. Tierney, Jr., S. J. McPhee, & M. A. Papadakis (Eds.), *Current medical diagnosis and treatment* (37th ed.). Stamford, CT: Appleton & Lange.

Griffin, D. E. (1997). Central nervous system infections. In J. D. Stobo, D. B. Hellmann, P. W. Ladenson, B. G. Petty, & T. A. Traill (Eds.), *The principles and practice of medicine* (23rd ed.). Stamford, CT: Appleton & Lange.

Shaw, J. C., Robertson, M, H., & Parker, F. (1996). Common skin disorders. In J. Noble (Ed.), *Textbook of primary care medicine* (2nd ed.). St. Louis: Mosby.

Neurological Disorders

Ruth M. Kleinpell

Select one best answer to the following questions.

1. The ACNP is performing an admitting history and physical examination on Harry P., a 34-year-old male, admitted for recent onset of seizures. He says that when he has a seizure he smells something burning, suddenly becomes unresponsive, then begins to stare and smack his lips. He is exhibiting signs and symptoms consistent with:

    a. Simple partial seizure
    b. Complex partial seizure
    c. Absence or petit mal seizure
    d. Secondary generalized partial seizure

2. A 42-year-old male with a history of epilepsy presents to the emergency room in status epilepticus. This type of seizure:

    a. Is not considered an emergency state until 20 minutes of seizure activity has occurred
    b. Increases cerebral oxygen requirements and decreases cerebral blood flow
    c. Can lead to hyperthermia, metabolic acidosis, and cardiovascular arrest
    d. Usually requires treatment with neuromuscular blockade agents

3. Ellen J. is a 32-year-old female who was diagnosed with myasthenia gravis four years ago. She presents to the emergency room with sudden onset of left ptosis, diplopia, dysphasia, and left extremity weakness. A tensilon test is performed and her symptoms immediately improve. She was most likely experiencing:

    a. Cholinergic crisis
    b. Thyrotoxicosis crisis
    c. Myasthenic crisis
    d. Acute transient ischemic attack

4. A 17-year-old male who sustained severe injuries in a motor vehicle accident begins to exhibit signs of the Cushing reflex in the ICU. The ACNP knows that Cushing's reflex indicates:

   a. Increased cerebral perfusion pressure
   b. Direct brain stem compression
   c. Worsening epidural hematoma
   d. Critical cerebral hypoxia

5. A one day postoperative craniotomy patient in the neurosurgical ICU begins to develop signs of increasing intracranial pressure (ICP). Which of the following measures would be effective in decreasing ICP?

   a. Increasing cerebral perfusion pressure
   b. Decreasing $PaCO_2$
   c. Increasing mean arterial pressure
   d. Decreasing PaO_2

6. Ken T., a 16-year-old male, is admitted for suspected meningitis. He has had an elevated temperature of 102° F for the past 24 hours prior to admission and reports a headache with nuchal rigidity. Which of the following would not be supportive of a diagnosis of meningitis?

   a. Presence of positive Kernig's sign
   b. Increased protein, glucose, and white blood cell (WBC) levels on lumbar puncture (LP)
   c. Positive Brudzinski's sign
   d. Cerebrospinal fluid (CSF) with elevated pressure

7. A 72-year-old female presents with a history of probable transient ischemic attacks (TIA). Which of the following is accurate with respect to TIA?

   a. It can be due to embolic or hemorrhagic etiologies
   b. It may result in cerebral infarction within five years in 50% of cases
   c. It is an indication for carotid artery endarterectomy with > 50% stenosis
   d. It can be treated with anticoagulant therapy to reverse thrombotic changes

8. Mr. B., a 69-year-old male, is in the emergency room with a sudden onset cerebrovascular accident (CVA). The incoming ACNP reviews all the assessment data that has been collected for this patient. Which of the following would not be a typical assessment finding?

   a. Ipsilateral pupil changes
   b. Contralateral motor changes such as weakness and paralysis

   c. Lumbar puncture with red blood cells (RBC) in the CSF
   d. Negative head computerized tomography (CT) scan

9. Seizure activity is classified into various categories depending upon symptoms and affected area of the brain. Which of the following is descriptive of simple partial seizures?

   a. The patient may have aura, staring and automatisms
   b. There is no loss of consciousness
   c. They are common in children and often involve rapid eye blinking
   d. They begin with tonic and progress to clonic contractions

10. Which of the following statements about tonic-clonic seizures is not correct?

   a. They are classified as generalized seizures
   b. An aura may occur followed by repetitive involuntary contractions
   c. They were previously known as grand mal seizures
   d. They can be subdivided into secondary generalized and absence or petit mal seizures

11. A 45-year-old male with a two week history of weakness is admitted to rule out myasthenia gravis. Which of the following statements is true with regard to myasthenia gravis?

   a. It results from demyelination of peripheral nerves
   b. It is classified as an autoimmune disorder
   c. It presents with an ascending muscle weakness progressing to paralysis
   d. It occurs due to a deficiency of acetylcholine at the neuromuscular junction

Questions 12 and 13 refer to the following scenario.

Mr. S. is a 39-year-old male presenting to the clinic with complaints of distal extremity paresthesias and leg stiffness for one week. He relates that two weeks ago he had a fever and an upper respiratory infection for which he did not seek medical treatment. He has bilateral lower leg weakness and hypoactive deep tendon reflexes (DTR).

12. The most likely diagnosis for Mr. S. is:

   a. Rheumatoid arthritis
   b. Myasthenia gravis

    c. Guillain-Barre

    d. Peripheral neuropathy

13. Based upon Mrs. S.'s presentation, the appropriate action would be to:

    a. Manage as an outpatient with a steroid taper

    b. Initiate antibiotic therapy

    c. Prepare for a lumbar puncture

    d. Hospitalize as flaccid paralysis can result

14. Ms. Z. is a 23-year-old female who presents to the emergency room with a two day history of headache, photophobia, nausea, vomiting, and fever. The differential diagnoses would include:

    a. Pituitary tumor

    b. Viral encephalopathy

    c. Meningitis

    d. Subarachnoid bleed

15. Encephalopathy is suspected in a confused elderly man. Which of the following statements is not correct with regard to encephalopathy?

    a. Symptoms depend on the cause and can range from headache to coma

    b. Encephalopathy is classified as a primary metabolic disease of the central nervous system (CNS)

    c. Cerebral function disturbances result from disease in another organ system

    d. Encephalopathy is considered an acquired metabolic disease of the CNS

16. Mr. S, a 17-year-old male, presents to the emergency room after being involved in a motor vehicle accident several hours ago. He is alert and oriented, moving all extremities freely, and denies any discomfort. A CT of the head is scheduled. The ACNP notes the presence of ecchymosis over the left mastoid area. This is indicative of:

    a. Fractured sinus bones

    b. Auditory canal hemorrhage

    c. Basilar skull fracture

    d. Epidural hematoma

17. MVA with resultant head trauma is a leading cause of morbidity in young adults. How does head trauma affect intracranial pressure?

    a. It increases CSF volume which maintains autoregulation and normalizes ICP

b. It results in an increase in cerebral perfusion pressure (CPP) which causes a decrease in ICP

c. It increases ICP as a compensatory response to acute volume loss

d. It has no effect on ICP unless a mass effect or intracranial hematoma occurs

18. A 43-year-old construction worker is admitted to the trauma unit after sustaining a 40 foot fall. He is intubated but is alert and follows commands. The results of magnetic resonance imaging (MRI) are pending. Upon physical examination, the ACNP finds loss of voluntary movement and proprioception with intact pain sensation to the left arm and leg, intact voluntary movement and proprioception but loss of pain sensation to the right arm and leg, fracture to the left arm, and suspected spinal cord injury. These findings are most consistent with:

a. Central cord syndrome

b. Cauda equina syndrome

c. Conus medularis syndrome

d. Brown-sequard syndrome

19. There are several neurological disorders with no firm diagnostic markers; diagnosis is often made clinically with supportive physical and laboratory findings. Which of the following is consistent with a diagnosis of Parkinson's disease?

a. It is a degenerative peripheral nervous system disorder

b. It results in excess production and impaired reuptake of dopamine

c. It often manifests with cogwheel rigidity, resting tremor, and bradykinesia

d. A ''pill-rolling'' tremor which can be lessened with cholinergic medications is characteristic

20. Mr. C., a 73-year-old male, was brought to the outpatient clinic by his neighbor after the neighbor noticed that Mr. C. had ''not been acting himself.'' Mr. C. currently has a temperature (temp) of 102° F, a blood pressure (BP) of 102/60 mm Hg, respiratory (resp) rate of 32 bpm, and heart rate of 104 bpm. He is disoriented and irritable but can follow commands. He is exhibiting signs and symptoms consistent with:

a. Confusion

b. Stupor

c. Dementia

d. Delirium

Answers and Rationale

1. **(b)** Complex partial seizure. Impaired level of consciousness, aura, staring, and automatisms, or repetitive, nonpurposeful movements are the presenting signs of a complex partial seizure. Complex partial seizures are often caused by benign lesions or an infarct in the temporal lobe (Graber, et al., p. 567).

2. **(c)** Status epilepticus is defined as a seizure of > 10 minutes duration, is considered an emergency state, and can lead to hyperthermia, metabolic acidosis and cardiovascular arrest. Status epilepticus increases cerebral oxygen requirements and increases cerebral blood flow. Parenteral anticonvulsants are used for treatment of seizures; barbiturate coma or general anesthesia with neuromuscular blockade may rarely be required when seizures persist (Carey, et al., p. 487).

3. **(c)** Myasthenic crisis. The tensilon test is used to differentiate myasthenic or cholinergic crisis in a patient diagnosed with myasthenia gravis. Edrophonium (tensilon) is an anticholinesterase inhibitor which produces a marked temporary improvement in muscle strength in myasthenic crisis. Symptoms worsen if the cause is due to cholinergic oversupply (Marino, pp. 797-799).

4. **(b)** Cushings reflex is a sign of direct brain stem compression that indicates cerebral perfusion pressure is not sufficient to meet oxygen requirements of the brain. A response of the cardiovascular system to increase blood flow, the triad of responses includes increased systolic blood pressure, bradycardia, and increased pulse pressure (Grodzin, et al., pp. 620).

5. **(d)** Mechanisms to decrease ICP include decreasing $PaCO_2$, increasing PaO_2, decreasing cerebral blood flow, and decreasing mean arterial pressure (Parsons & Wiener-Kronish, pp. 348-354).

6. **(b)** Findings suggestive of meningitis include the presence of a positive Kernig's and Brudzinski's sign, increased protein, decreased glucose, the presence of WBC on lumbar puncture, and CSF with elevated pressure (Grodzin, et al., pp. 281-286).

7. **(a)** Transient ischemic attacks can be due to embolic or hemorrhagic etiologies. 30% of patients will have a cerebral infarction within five years. A stenosis > 70% is an indication for carotid artery endarterectomy. Antithrombolytic therapy may be used to reverse vessel occlusions (American Heart Association, pp. 835; Carey, et al., pp. 483-485).

8. **(c)** Lumbar puncture is contraindicated with cerebrovascular infarcts as brain stem herniation can be induced with rapid decompression of the subarachnoid space (Carey, et al., pp. 484).

9. **(b)** Simple partial seizures have no loss of consciousness and often involve motor symptoms frequently starting in a single muscle group and spreading to an entire side of the body. Paresthesias, flashing lights, vocalizations and hallucinations are common manifestations of simple partial seizures (Graber, et al., pp. 567).

10. **(d)** Tonic-clonic seizures and absence or petit mal seizures are two subcategories of generalized seizures (Graber, et al., pp. 567).

11. **(b)** Myasthenia gravis is an autoimmune disorder of the neuromuscular junction resulting in a reduction of the number of acetylcholine receptor sites at the neuromuscular junction. Muscle weakness results from impaired impulse transmission. The weakness is typically worse after exercise and better after rest, but constant weakness may occur. The clinical course is variable with spontaneous remissions and exacerbations and treatment is based on symptoms (Carey, et al., pp. 491-492).

12. **(c)** Guillain-Barre is an inflammatory process of the nervous system characterized by demyelination of peripheral nerves resulting in progressive, symmetrical, ascending paralysis. Although the cause is unknown, the syndrome is usually preceded by a suspected viral infection accompanied by fever 1 to 3 weeks before the onset of acute bilateral muscle weakness in the lower extremities (Carey, et al., p. 490).

13. **(d)** The presentation of Guillain-Barre is typically a rapidly progressive, ascending paralysis. Flaccid paralysis can result within 48 to 72 hours as autodigestion of the myelin sheath occurs. Hospitalization is required as respi-

ratory function must be monitored closely and mechanical ventilation is often needed (Carey, et al., p. 490).

14. **(c)** Meningitis should be considered in any patient with fever and neurologic symptoms. Acute bacterial meningitis is a medical emergency and prognosis depends on the interval between onset of disease and the initiation of antibiotics (Grodzin, et al., pp. 281-286).

15. **(b)** Encephalopathy is an acquired or secondary metabolic disease of the nervous system (Fauci, et al., pp. 2451-2453).

16. **(c)** Ecchymosis over the mastoid area, called Battle's sign, is indicative of a basilar skull fracture (Parsons & Wiener-Kronish, p. 350).

17. **(c)** Head trauma increases ICP. As the cranium is a fixed space composed of brain tissue, blood, and CSF, a change in the volume of any one must result in a compensatory change in another. In head trauma, an increase in mass due to cerebral edema or hematoma occurs. Physiologic compensatory mechanisms are transient, and a rise in ICP occurs with head trauma (Marino, p. 814).

18. **(d)** Brown-Sequard syndrome is an incomplete spinal cord injury. The injured side displays loss of voluntary movement and proprioception but intact pain sensation, and the opposite side displays voluntary movement and proprioception but loss of pain sensation. Central cord syndrome results from injury to centrally located spinal cord tracts. Movement and sensation may be present in the lower extremities but not in the upper. Cauda equina syndrome results from compression of lower lumbar and sacral roots. Lower extremity paralysis, sensory loss, and bladder and rectal dysfunction can result. A second type of lumbar and sacral root injury is conus medularis syndrome which results in lower leg weakness, impaired bowel and bladder and sensory loss in the "saddle" area of the perineum (Carey, et al., p. 402).

19. **(c)** Parkinson's disease is progressive, degenerative central nervous system disorder which results in an imbalance of dopamine and acetycholine in the

striatum. Characteristic signs include cogwheel rigidity, resting or "pill-rolling" tremor, bradykinesia or slowness of movement, and postural reflex instability. Pharmacologic intervention is aimed at restoring the balance or loss of dopamine, often with a combination medication containing levodopa, the precursor to dopamine, and carbidopa, an inhibitor of an enzyme that prevents peripheral breakdown of dopamine (Graber, et al., pp 569-575).

20. **(d)** Delirium refers to an abnormal mental state characterized by disorientation, fear, irritability and misperception of sensory stimuli. Delirium often results from drugs, fever, and sepsis. Confusion describes a state of inattentiveness that is characterized by misinterpretation of sensory stimuli, faulty memory, bewilderment, and difficulty following commands. Stupor is a state where the level of consciousness is depressed but from which the patient can be aroused by vigorous and repeated stimuli. Dementia refers to a deterioration of intellectual function without diminution of arousal. Impairment of higher cortical functioning memory, language, calculation, attention and orientation occurs with dementia (Grodzin, et al., p. 629).

References

American Heart Association. (1996). Guidelines for the management of transient ischemic attacks. *Neurology, 47,* 835.

Carey, C., Lee, H., & Woeltje, K. (1998). *The Washington manual of medical therapeutics.* Philadelphia: Lippincott-Raven.

Fauci, A., Braunwald, E., Isselbacher, K., Wilson, J., Martin, J., Kasper, D., Hauser, S., & Longo, D. (1998). *Harrison's principles of internal medicine.* (14th ed.). NY: McGraw-Hill.

Graber, M., Toth, P., & Herting, R. (1997). *The family practice handbook.* St. Louis: Mosby.

Grodzin, C., Schwartz, S., & Bone, R. (1996). *Diagnostic strategies for internal medicine.* St. Louis: Mosby.

Marino, P. (1998). *The ICU book* (2nd ed.). Baltimore: Williams & Wilkins.

Parsons, P., & Wiener-Kronish, J. (1998). *Critical care secrets.* St. Louis: Mosby.

Respiratory Disorders

Lynn A. Kelso

Select one best answer to the following questions.

1. A 36-year-old, 72 kg female, intubated for a severe asthma exacerbation, is on the following ventilator settings: Tidal volume (V_T) 650 mL; simultaneous intermittent mandatory ventilation (SIMV) rate 14; fraction of inspired oxygen (FiO_2) 0.75. Her morning arterial blood gas (ABG) was: pH 7.08; $PaCO_2$ 55 mm Hg; PaO_2 88 mm Hg; HCO_3^- 21 mEq/L. Which of the following orders is appropriate in response to this ABG?

   a. Increase V_T to 700 mL
   b. Increase SIMV rate to 18
   c. Decrease FiO_2 to 0.50
   d. Administer 2 amps $NaHCO_3$ IV

2. You are called to evaluate a 22-year-old male who presents to the emergency department secondary to an exacerbation of his asthma. When you arrive the patient is lethargic but oriented with a BP of 116/82 mm Hg, heart rate 64 bpm, resp 36 bpm, and temp 37.2° C. The ABG includes a pH of 7.32, $PaCO_2$ of 42 mm Hg, and PaO_2 of 82 mm Hg on 4L O_2 via nasal cannula. The most appropriate action would be to:

   a. Administer albuterol and admit to the floor
   b. Administer albuterol, prednisone, and admit to the ICU
   c. Administer inhaled cromolyn sulfate, albuterol, and reassess in 60 minutes
   d. Admit to the floor for continued observation

3. When evaluating an asthmatic patient's respiratory status, which parameter is the best indicator of a severe exacerbation?

   a. Peak expiratory flow < 80% of personal best
   b. Forced vital capacity < 80% of predicted
   c. Peak expiratory flow < 50% of personal best
   d. Forced vital capacity < 50% of predicted

Questions 4 and 5 refer to the following scenario.

A 74-year-old male who had a pelvic abscess drainage five days ago is complaining of chest pain and shortness of breath. His current vital signs are as follows: BP 90/56 mm Hg; heart rate 118 bpm; resp 28 bpm. He is afebrile with a pulse oximeter reading of 93% on 4L O_2 via nasal cannula. His past medical history is significant only for prostate cancer. On physical examination he is anxious but alert and oriented, heart sounds are normal, and bilateral breath sounds are remarkable for diffuse inspiratory crackles.

4. Your initial orders should include:

   a. 50% O_2, heparin 5000 units IV, ECG
   b. 50% O_2, posterior/anterior (PA) and lateral chest radiograph
   c. 30% O_2, heparin 3000 units IV, echocardiogram
   d. 50% O_2, ECG, serial cardiac enzymes

5. The above patient, who is 83 kg, is emergently intubated for respiratory failure. The most appropriate initial ventilator settings are:

   a. V_T 600 mL; FiO_2 0.40; RR 12; PEEP 5 cm H_2O
   b. V_T 600 mL; FiO_2 1.0; RR 18; PEEP 5 cm H_2O
   c. V_T 800 mL; FiO_2 0.80; RR 12; PEEP 5 cm H_2O
   d. V_T 1000 mL; FiO_2 1.0; RR 12; PEEP 5 cm H_2O

Questions 6, 7, and 8 refer to the following scenario.

A 69-year-old female patient was admitted for a laparoscopic cholecystectomy. 24 hours after her procedure she has a temperature of 38.9° C, heart rate of 109 bpm, resp of 28 bpm, and BP of 102/74 mm Hg. Her chest radiograph shows an infiltrate of the right upper lobe. Physical examination reveals diffuse crackles and she has a cough productive of white sputum.

6. After obtaining blood and sputum cultures you order empiric antibiotics. Which of the following is the most appropriate antibiotic choice?

   a. Ceftriaxone 1 gm IV q12h
   b. Cefuroxime 250 mg p.o. b.i.d.
   c. Gentamicin 5 mg/kg IV q.d.
   d. Ciprofloxacin 400 mg IV q.d.

7. 72 hours after the initiation of antibiotics the above patient has the following vital signs: BP 92/64 mm Hg; heart rate 121 bpm; resp 24 bpm; temp 39.1° C.

Sputum production has increased and oxygen saturation (SaO_2) is 90% on 4L O_2 via nasal cannula. In response to these clinical signs the most appropriate action would be to:

   a. Repeat blood and sputum cultures and increase the current antibiotic regimen
   b. Consult pulmonary for a fiberoptic bronchoscopy and order an aminoglycoside
   c. Begin amphotericin B with goal of 0.5 mg/kg/d
   d. Consult surgery for an open lung biopsy and order erythromycin 500 mg IV q6h.

8. The above patient develops a large pleural effusion seen on chest radiograph. A diagnostic tap reveals clear, pale yellow fluid with a pH of 7.02, glucose of 24 mg/dL, and lactic dehydrogenase (LDH) of 1924 IU/L. The cell count is RBC 263/µL, WBC 21,342/µL with 73% polymorphonucleocytes (PMN) and 12% monocytes. The best course of action would be:

   a. Chest tube placement to drain the effusion
   b. Drainage of the effusion for symptomatic relief
   c. Serial chest radiographs to follow the extent of the effusion
   d. Drainage of 500 cc to send for cytology

9. A 43-year-old female is suspected of having tuberculosis. While awaiting the sputum cultures the best medication regimen is:

   a. Isoniazid (INH), rifampin
   b. INH, rifampin, pyrazinamide
   c. INH, streptomycin, ethambutol
   d. INH, rifampin, pyrazinamide, streptomycin

Questions 10 and 11 refer to the following scenario.

A 73-year-old male is admitted to your service with increased cough and increased production of thick, yellow sputum. His past medical history is significant for COPD, and he has a 57 pack year smoking history.

10. You suspect infection as the cause of his problems. Empiric antibiotic therapy should cover:

   a. *Candida albicans*
   b. *Pseudomonas aeruginosa*

c. *Streptococcus pneumoniae*
d. *Chlamydia pneumoniae*

11. Upon admission a patient's ABG reveals a pH of 7.36, $PaCO_2$ of 59 mm Hg, PaO_2 of 49 mm Hg, and HCO_3^- of 29 mEq/L on 2L O_2 via nasal cannula. The patient is anxious and sitting on the edge of the bed. He has circumoral cyanosis, and lung fields auscultate for expiratory wheezes bilaterally. The ACNP should order:

    a. Lorazepam 2 mg IV
    b. Albuterol 2 puffs q2-4h
    c. Prednisone 60 mg q6h
    d. 60% O_2 via face mask

Questions 12 and 13 refer to the following scenario.

A 48-year-old female is in the ICU with acute pancreatitis. Her vital signs are as follows: BP 92/60 mm Hg; heart rate 116 bpm; central venous pressure (CVP) 9 mm Hg; pulmonary artery pressure (PAP) 29/18 mm Hg; pulmonary capillary wedge pressure (PCWP) 14 mm Hg. She is intubated with current ventilator settings of V_T 800 mL, assist control (AC) rate 14 bpm, FiO_2 0.85, and positive end expiratory pressure (PEEP) 5.0 cm H_2O. Her ABG reveals a pH of 7.31, $PaCO_2$ of 48 mm Hg, and a PaO_2 of 62 mm Hg. Her chest radiograph shows diffuse, fluffy infiltrates.

12. Based upon this assessment the ACNP would order:

    a. An increase of FiO_2 to 0.95
    b. An increase of PEEP to 7.5 cm H_2O
    c. An increase of rate to 18 bpm
    d. An increase of V_T to 900 mL

13. The patient's peak airway pressures are now 45 mm Hg. The next appropriate action would be to:

    a. Have a chest tube kit placed at the best side
    b. Change to volume-control ventilation
    c. Paralyze and sedate the patient
    d. Change to pressure-control ventilation

Questions 14 and 15 refer to the following scenario.

A 21-year-old male is admitted with dyspnea and left sided chest pain which woke him during the night. He has been experiencing the same pain for 48 hours and sought medical attention because he was unable to complete basketball practice.

14. The diagnostic test which would be most helpful in this situation is a(n):

   a. ECG
   b. Chest radiograph
   c. Echocardiogram
   d. Chest CT scan

15. The ACNP decides to admit the patient. Admission orders must include:

   a. Cefuroxime 250 mg p.o. b.i.d.
   b. Bedrest, with q.a.m. ECG
   c. Bedrest, with chest radiograph in 12 hours
   d. Fiberoptic bronchoscopy

16. Prior to surgery, an asthmatic patient should have:

   a. A course of oral steroids
   b. Pulmonary function tests
   c. A three day course of increased β_2 agonists
   d. Empiric antibiotic therapy

17. When doing a preoperative assessment on a 37-year-old asthmatic, it is important to have information related to which of the following:

   a. Hospitalizations within the previous year
   b. Arterial blood gas analysis
   c. Ventilator days within the previous six months
   d. Systemic corticosteroid use in the previous six months

Questions 18 and 19 refer to the following scenario.

A 23-year-old male is admitted with shortness of breath, hemoptysis, and fever. His temp is 38.3° C, BP 116/84 mm Hg, heart rate 108 bpm, and resp 20 bpm. His chest radiograph shows a left upper lobe infiltrate.

18. Admission orders should include which of the following?

   a. Sputum gram stain on admission
   b. Respiratory isolation
   c. Oral corticosteroids
   d. IV antibiotics

19. In addition to routine admission laboratory studies the ACNP should order:

    a. HIV screening
    b. CK with isoenzymes
    c. ECG
    d. Chest CT

20. A 32-year-old male patient is complaining of difficulty swallowing. His temperature is 38.6° C. On physical examination he has cervical adenopathy and his pharynx is inflamed with visible exudate. His rapid antigen test was negative. The appropriate action would be to:

    a. Discharge to home
    b. Order p.o. erythromycin
    c. Order IV ampicillin
    d. Repeat rapid antigen test in 24 hours

Answers and Rationale

1. **(d)** Asthmatic patients who require intubation for severe exacerbation should be treated with IV sodium bicarbonate for respiratory acidosis. Permissive hypercapnia is the recommended ventilatory strategy. The goal is to provide adequate oxygenation for the patient while minimizing high airway pressures and consequently the risk of barotrauma (NIH Guidelines, p. 67).

2. **(b)** Impending signs of respiratory failure include bradycardia, tachypnea, and absence of wheezing. Respiratory drive is typically increased with asthma exacerbations so a normal $PaCO_2$ indicates an increased risk of respiratory failure. Also, with the patient lethargic, a further alteration in mental status may necessitate intubation (Pittman, p. 219).

3. **(c)** Peak expiratory flow should be measured regularly. A PEF < 80% of the patient's personal best, prior to bronchodilator use, indicates a need for increased medications. A PEF < 50% of personal best indicates a severe exacerbation (NIH Guidelines, p. 16).

4. **(a)** These symptoms are consistent with pulmonary embolism. Initial therapy should include an increase in FiO_2 in order to provide adequate oxygenation. An ECG should be done in order to rule out cardiac involvement. As long as there are no absolute contraindications, heparin should be started immediately based upon clinical suspicion (Schuller, p. 204).

5. **(c)** When initiating ventilator settings, a physiologic respiratory rate and higher FiO_2 should be used. An approximate estimation for tidal volume is 10 mL/kg. Further ventilator settings can be based upon arterial blood gas analysis (Kollef, p. 178).

6. **(a)** The patient has symptoms consistent with pneumonia. Hospital acquired pneumonia is considered to occur after 48 hours. Since the patient has only been hospitalized for 24 hours, community acquired pneumonia should be suspected. The most common pathogens are *S. pneumoniae, H. influenzae, S. aureus,* respiratory viruses, or aerobic gram negative bacilli. Although either ceftriaxone or cefuroxime could be used, it is recommended that patients over the age of 60 who are hospitalized receive IV antibiotics (Stauffer, p. 279).

7. **(b)** Because the patient's condition has worsened on IV antibiotics, further diagnostic tests are required. Fiberoptic bronchoscopy is the best option presented. The patient has now been hospitalized long enough to develop a hospital acquired pneumonia, and an aminoglycoside could be added to cephalosporin therapy (Stauffer, p. 281).

8. **(a)** A pH of < 7.10, glucose of < 40 mg/dL, and LDH > 1,000 IU/L indicates a complicated parapneumonic effusion. Patients who have a complicated effusion should have complete drainage of the effusion which may require the placement of a chest tube (Schuller, p. 193).

9. **(d)** Initial therapy of uncomplicated tuberculosis should include four drugs unless there is very little risk of drug resistance. Once culture and sensitivity reports are received, drug therapy can be tailored to resistance. It is also important to know the drug resistance patterns where the patient lives (Mundy, p. 279).

10. **(c)** In acute exacerbations of COPD, the most common organisms are *Streptococcus pneumoniae, Haemophilus influenzae,* and *Mycoplasma pneumoniae* (Schuller, p. 195).

11. **(d)** Oxygen should be administered in order to keep the PaO_2 between 55 and 65 mm/Hg. This should be done despite the possibility of hypercapnia. Although albuterol would be appropriate, the dose given in the response is not adequate for an exacerbation (Schuller, p. 195).

12. **(b)** This patient is at risk for developing ARDS secondary to her pancreatitis. Because of her low filling pressures, it is not likely that she is experiencing cardiogenic pulmonary edema. In order to improve oxygenation, increasing PEEP is most beneficial. Increasing the FiO_2 will increase the risk of oxygen toxicity and you will gain no oxygenation benefit from increasing the rate or the tidal volume (Marino, pp. 376-381).

13. **(d)** In order to decrease the risk of lung injury, there is a need to decrease peak inspiratory pressures. This is best accomplished by using a pressure-control ventilation mode which will set a maximal pressure limit and also deliver an adequate tidal volume. The patient will require sedation because this mode is not well tolerated in patients who are awake, but may not require paralysis (Marino, pp. 381, 438).

14. **(b)** This patient has indications of a spontaneous pneumothorax. Patients are usually young and the acute onset of ipsilateral chest pain and dyspnea is often of several days duration by the time medical attention is sought. The most important diagnostic examination would be a chest radiograph which would show evidence of air in the pleural space (Stauffer, pp. 330-331).

15. **(c)** Treatment is based upon the severity of the pneumothorax. Patients who present with a new small pneumothorax should be hospitalized and placed on bedrest. Evaluation of the patient should include chest radiographs every 12 to 24 hours. If there is any deterioration in the patient's condition, placement of a chest tube should be considered (Stauffer, p. 331).

16. **(b)** Asthmatic patients should have an assessment of pulmonary function prior to elective surgery (NIH Guidelines, p. 56).

17. **(d)** Patients who have been on systemic corticosteroids for longer than two weeks, within six months prior to surgery, should receive hydrocortisone 100 mg IV every eight hours during the surgical period (NIH Guidelines, p. 56).

18. **(b)** This patient has symptoms suggestive of tuberculosis. Patients who present with symptoms that may indicate tuberculosis should be placed on respiratory isolation until tuberculosis is ruled out. A sputum gram stain is not adequate and a sputum for acid fast bacilli (AFB) needs to be ordered. This patient has no indications for steroids. While you may choose to begin antibiotics, they are not the best choice for TB (Mundy, p. 279).

19. **(a)** Young patients are not frequently infected with tuberculosis unless there is a compromised immune system. HIV status should be assessed on these patients so that appropriate treatment measures can be undertaken if the patient is HIV positive (Stauffer, p. 283).

20. **(b)** These symptoms are classic for pharyngitis caused by *Streptococcus pyogenes*. Because 15% of these infections can lead to serious complications, they do need to be treated. The rapid antigen test is specific but lacks sensitivity. Therefore, if the test is positive you may begin treatment, but if the test is negative you must treat and wait until the culture comes back negative to confirm the absence of infection (Durand, p. 183).

References

Durand, M., Joseph, M., & Baker, A. S. (1998). Infections of the upper respiratory tract. In A. S. Fauci, E. Braunwald, K. J. Isselbacher, J. D. Wilson, J. B. Martin, D. L. Kasper, S. L. Hauser, & D. L. Longo (Eds.), *Harrison's principles of internal medicine* (14th ed., pp. 179-184). NY: McGraw-Hill.

Kollef, M. H. (1998). Critical care. In C. F. Carey, H. H. Lee, & K. F. Woeltje (Eds.), *The Washington manual of medical therapeutics* (29th ed., pp. 170-189). Philadelphia: Lippincott-Raven.

Highlights of the expert panel report #2. *Guidelines for the diagnosis and management of asthma.* (1997). National Institutes of Health/National Heart, Lung and Blood Institute. Publication #97-4051a.

Marino, P. L. (1998). *The ICU book* (2nd ed.). Baltimore: Williams & Wilkins.

Mundy, L. M., & L'Ecuyer, P. B. (1998). Treatment of infectious diseases. In C. F. Carey, H. H. Lee, & K. F. Woeltje (Eds.), *The Washington manual of medical therapeutics* (29th ed., pp. 260-287). Philadelphia: Lippincott-Raven.

Pittman, A., & Tillinghast, J. (1998). Allergy and immunlogy. In C. F. Carey, H. H. Lee, & K. F. Woeltje (Eds.), *The Washington manual of medical therapeutics* (29th ed., pp. 213-226). Philadelphia: Lippincott-Raven.

Schuller, D. (1998). Pulmonary diseases. In C. F. Carey, H. H. Lee, & K. F. Woeltje (Eds.), *The Washington manual of medical therapeutics* (29th ed., pp. 190-212). Philadelphia: Lippincott-Raven.

Stauffer, J. L. (1998). Lung. In L. M. Tierney, Jr., S. J. McPhee, & M. A. Papadakis (Eds.), *Current medical diagnosis and treatment* (37th ed., pp. 251-332). Stamford, CT: Appleton & Lange.

Cardiovascular Disorders

Candis Morrison

Select one best answer to the following questions.

Questions 1 and 2 refer to the following scenario.

A 62-year-old male presents with complaints of lightheadedness and fatigue of 20 minutes duration. He reports similar episodes occurring over the past two weeks. On examination he is slightly anxious. Vital signs are as follows: Temp 36.5° C, heart rate 50 bpm, resp 18 bpm, and BP 100/80 mm Hg. The chest is clear to auscultation. ECG analysis shows no discrete P waves and irregular atrial activity of > 350 bpm. Ventricular rate is irregular, however no ventricular ectopic beats are noted. This rhythm is confirmed in multiple leads.

1. This clinical picture is most consistent with which rhythm?

    a. Atrial flutter
    b. Atrial fibrillation
    c. Ventricular fibrillation
    d. Ventricular ectopy

2. The treatment goals for this patient include:

    a. Control of the atrial rate and thrombolytic therapy
    b. Decreased cardiac output and anxiolytic therapy
    c. Increased coronary artery perfusion and decreased oxygen demand
    d. Increased atrio-ventricular (AV) node conduction and decreased international ratio (INR)

Questions 3 and 4 refer to the following scenario.

A 64-year-old male is brought into the emergency department with a chief complaint of substernal chest pressure for the past 30 minutes. This is associated with nausea and diaphoresis. He has a history of angina, which was previously relieved with nitroglycerin (NTG). He is a 30 pack year smoker. He has had three tablets of sublingual (SL) NTG but the pain persists. Physical examination reveals a heart rate of 80 bpm, resp of 30 bpm, and BP of 104/60 mm Hg. The ECG demonstrates ST segment elevation in leads II, III, and aVF.

3. Based on these symptoms and findings, which wall of the heart do you suspect is affected?

   a. Anterior
   b. Lateral
   c. Posterior
   d. Inferior

4. He is transferred to the cardiac care unit (CCU) where thrombolytic therapy is initiated. His chest pain is relieved. An additional sign of successful reperfusion would be:

   a. Return of CK enzymes to normal values
   b. Normal ventricular ejection fraction
   c. Return of ST segment to baseline
   d. T wave inversion in leads II, III and aVF

Questions 5 and 6 refer to the following scenario.

A 79-year-old post acute MI patient has been in the CCU for three days. She now reports constant pain which worsens with deep inspiration. She says she is most comfortable leaning forward in her bed. Vital signs include a heart rate of 112 bpm, resp of 24 bpm, and BP of 130/79 mm Hg. The ECG demonstrates nonspecific ST segment changes.

5. What is most likely the cause of these signs and symptoms?

   a. Costochondritis
   b. Pneumonia
   c. Pericardial tamponade
   d. Pericarditis

6. Later that night, the patient develops sudden hypotension, her BP drops to 80/50 mm Hg and her heart rate elevates to 130 bpm. Upon physical examination you observe jugular vein distention (JVD) and auscultate muffled heart sounds and pulsus paradoxus. Which complication should be suspected?

a. Pulmonary embolism
b. Ventricular septal rupture
c. Ruptured papillary muscle
d. Cardiac tamponade

7. An 88-year-old patient is admitted from the nursing home in acute congestive heart failure (CHF). Nursing home staff reports that his normal weight is 71 kg. Upon admission his vital signs include a heart rate of 104 bpm, resp of 28 bpm, and BP of 120/60 mm Hg. His weight is 73.5 kg. Cardiovascular examination reveals regular rate and rhythm. There are crackles in both lung bases. After several hours in the intensive care unit he becomes increasingly short of breath and you hear an S_3 at the apex. His BP has decreased to 80/60 mm Hg and his heart rate has risen to 130 bpm. He is breathing 40 times per minute. Your immediate treatment goals are to:

   a. Reduce preload and afterload
   b. Reduce afterload and contractility
   c. Reduce preload and improve contractility
   d. Reduce afterload and improve contractility

8. Which pharmacotherapeutic agents would you select to achieve these goals in this patient?

   a. Dobutamine and furosemide
   b. Dobutamine and nitroprusside
   c. Morphine sulfate and nitroprusside
   d. Furosemide and MSO$_4$

9. Which of the following categories of medications are used in CHF patients to block a maladaptive compensatory mechanism?

   a. Cardiac glycosides
   b. Angiotensin converting enzyme (ACE) inhibitors
   c. Vasodilators
   d. Diuretics

10. A 42-year-old female reports to the urgent care center complaining that she failed to refill her BP medication prescription and now she has a severe, throbbing, occipital headache. Her BP is 200/120 mm Hg. She is transferred to the emergency department where oxygen is started simultaneously with intravenous access. The next step in her care would be to administer:

   a. Vasodilators to decrease preload

    b. Inotropes to increase contractility

    c. Beta blockers to control heart rate

    d. Analgesics to provide pain relief

11. A temporary transvenous ventricular pacemaker is inserted into a 65-year-old patient in 3rd degree heart block. Immediately following the procedure his heart rate is 80 bpm. Two hours later he states that he is increasingly dizzy, despite the fact that he is supine in bed. His systolic blood pressure is 80 mm Hg and his ventricular rate per monitor is 48 bpm. No pacing spikes are evident. This means that:

    a. There is failure to capture and return to the intrinsic rhythm

    b. There is failure to pace and return to the intrinsic rhythm

    c. There is failure to sense and return to the intrinsic rhythm

    d. The pacemaker is competing with the intrinsic rhythm

12. When counseling a 40-year-old female with a cholesterol of 260 mg/dL about dietary modifications, a step 1 diet is prescribed. A desired outcome of this treatment is:

    a. A high density lipoprotein (HDL) cholesterol level < 50 mg/dL

    b. A cholesterol level decrease of 15% to 20%

    c. A triglyceride level between 200 mg/dL and 300 mg/dL.

    d. A low density lipoprotein (LDL) cholesterol level >115 mg/dL

13. A 60-year-old patient is brought to the emergency department with a history of severe substernal chest pain. It has not been relieved with three doses of nitroglycerin 0.5 mg and 25 mg of MSO_4 (cumulative). During examination the patient is diaphoretic and anxious. Her BP is 170/100 mm Hg in the right arm and 90/60 mm Hg in the left. Femoral pulses are barely palpable, and her feet are mottled. Chest radiograph reveals a widened mediastinum and a calcified aortic knob. This clinical picture is consistent with:

    a. Cardiac tamponade

    b. Acute pulmonary edema

    c. Pulmonary embolism

    d. Dissecting aortic aneurysm

14. H.B. is a 48-year-old patient followed by the ACNP for management of chronic hypertension and dyslipidemia. He also has a 40 pack year smoking history. He recently developed a new S_4 on physical examination. There are no murmurs or rubs. His chest is clear to auscultation. A new S_4 should alert the ACNP to the possibility of which of the following?

a. Pericarditis
b. Left bundle branch block
c. Acute MI
d. Cardiomyopathy

15. A 38-year-old patient is brought into the emergency department in complete cardiopulmonary arrest. Cardiopulmonary rescusitation (CPR) was initiated within four minutes in the field and maintained during transport. Two large bore intravenous accesses were also started before transport. The monitor shows asystole. Which drug does the American Heart Association deem first line (1A) therapy for this situation?

a. Atropine
b. Dopamine
c. Lidocaine
d. Epinephrine

16. A 47-year-old patient is placed on the monitor in the emergency department. It shows polymorphic ventricular tachycardia and a prolonged QT interval. This patient's medication history includes amitriptyline for several years. Which agent is used to treat this particular dysrhythmia?

a. Magnesium sulfate
b. Digitalis
c. Diuretics
d. MSO_4

17. S.L. is a 68-year-old male with aortic stenosis. In addition to chest pain, which of the following would indicate an urgent need for aortic valve replacement?

a. Aortic calcification
b. Left ventricular hypertrophy
c. Pulmonary hypertension
d. Syncope

18. A 28-year-old patient presents with history of cough, dyspnea, arthralgias and a fever of 10 days duration. Past medical history is negative for heart disease or murmur. Social history reveals that he has used intravenous drugs for the past two years. Upon physical examination his temperature is 38.8° C and there is a grade III systolic murmur at the left sternal border. You note subungual hemorrhages and erythematous lesions on the palms and soles. Abdominal examination reveals splenomegaly, but no masses. This history and clinical picture is strongly suggestive of:

    a. Pericarditis
    b. Endocarditis
    c. Pericardial effusion
    d. Pulmonary embolus

19. When performing hypertension screening on a new patient you determine that the right arm BP is 150/98 mm Hg. No other abnormalities are found. It is important to remember that:

    a. Hypertension may be diagnosed with a single elevated reading if it is in excess of 150/95 mm Hg
    b. Hypertension is diagnosed after three consecutive readings >140/90 mm Hg
    c. Hypertension of this magnitude requires institution of pharmacologic therapy
    d. Hypertension of this magnitude is of no concern and the patient can be re-assured

20. You are anticipating weaning your patient from the intra-aortic balloon pump that was inserted post coronary bypass surgery. Which are the two most important monitoring parameters to consider before beginning the weaning process?

    a. Cardiac index and systemic vascular resistance
    b. Systemic vascular resistance and pulmonary artery wedge pressure
    c. Cardiac index and mean arterial pressure
    d. Mean arterial pressure and pulmonary artery wedge pressure

Answers and Rationale

1. **(b)** This clinical and electrocardiographic picture is consistent with atrial fibrillation. In atrial fibrillation the atrial rate is in excess of 350 bpm and is difficult to calculate. The ventricular rate may be low. R to R intervals are irregular. P waves are indistinguishable. The atria are contracting rapidly and are thus unable to refill before ejection. The ventricles are filled inadequately and cardiac output is diminished, producing the symptoms described. There is an irregular ventricular response and there is a difference between the apical heart rate and the peripheral pulse rate (Kidd, pp. 270-272).

2. **(a)** Acute treatment of atrial fibrillation addresses the issues of rate control (per delivery of an IV agent that slows conduction across the AV node) and prevention of thromboembolic complications as atrial fibrillation of > 24 hours duration increases the risk of this phenomenon. In patients over 60-years-old, the risk of embolization warrants anticoagulation (Wang & Estes, pp. 83-85).

3. **(d)** Leads II, III, and aVF all have their positive leads at the foot and are looking up at the inferior aspect of the heart. Inferior wall myocardial infarctions are often associated with nausea (Ferri, p. 214).

4. **(c)** Successful reperfusion with thrombolytic therapy is demonstrated by abrupt cessation of chest pain and decrease in ST segment elevation (Lilly, pp. 324-235).

5. **(d)** Pericarditis is an inflammatory process that develops in up to 15% of patients 2 to 7 days postacute myocardial infarction. Nonspecific ST segment changes indicate generalized injury to the myocardium. Pain of pericarditis is typically best tolerated by leaning forward in the sitting position (Lilly, pp. 233, 242).

6. **(d)** Patients with pericarditis are especially susceptible to cardiac tamponade. Effusion develops in the pericardium and presses on the heart chambers. Classic signs are sinus tachycardia, hypotension, pulsus paradoxus, and electrical alternans (Roberts, pp. 117-119).

7. **(c)** This patient exhibits signs and symptoms of acute left CHF. The goals for this patient are to decrease preload to decrease cardiac work, and to improve contractility to optimize heart function (Kimmelsteil & Konstam, pp. 57-64).

8. **(a)** Dobutamine and furosemide would achieve the treatment goals. Dobutamine has positive inotropic effects on the heart that optimize cardiac output through increasing contractility. Furosemide, as a diuretic, will decrease cardiac work via its effect on decreasing preload. Nitroprusside would decrease BP excessively, as would MSO_4 (Kimmelstiel & Konstam, p. 67).

9. **(b)** ACE inhibitors will block a maladaptive compensatory mechanism in CHF. Renin is secreted by the kidney in response to decreased glomerular filtration rate. Renin causes conversion of angiotensinogen to angiotensin I which is then converted to angiotensin II by ACE as it passes through the lungs. Angiotensin II is a potent vasoconstrictor that also causes release of aldosterone from the adrenal cortex. Aldosterone causes the kidney to retain Na^+ and water and excrete K^+. This compensatory mechanism is adaptive in shock but maladaptive in CHF. ACE inhibitors block the conversion of angiotensin I to II preventing the increase in afterload caused by the vasoconstrictive effects of angiotensin II, and thus prevent increase in preload caused by Na^+ and water retention effects of aldosterone (Kimmelstiel & Konstam, pp. 69-70).

10. **(a)** This patient presents with a hypertensive urgency, and BP must be reduced within a few hours. Parenteral therapy is rarely required and partial reduction of blood pressure with relief of symptoms is the goal. The goal of therapy is to decrease preload. Vasodilators will achieve this goal (Massie, p. 445).

11. **(b)** Failure to pace is evidenced by a lack of pacing spikes on the monitor or ECG. When this occurs, the rhythm resorts to the prepacemaker rhythm (Dirks, pp. 182-184).

12. **(b)** Restriction of saturated fats and dietary cholesterol are the mainstay of dietary treatment of hyperlipidemia. In the first phase of treatment (step 1), saturated fat is restricted to 10% of total calories and dietary cholesterol to 300 mg/d. Ideally, this will lead to a decrease in serum cholesterol of 15% to 20% (Baron, p. 1144).

13. **(d)** This is a classic dissecting aneurysm. It can be differentiated from an MI or a pulmonary embolism by the chest radiograph findings and the BP discrepancies (Tierney & Messina, pp. 451-452).

14. **(c)** This patient has multiple risk factors for acute myocardial infarction. An S_4 is associated with a noncompliant ventricle, which occurs in myocardial infarction and left ventricular hypertrophy (Lilly, p. 234).

15. **(d)** Epinephrine is first line therapy in a pulseless situation. Atropine would be second line. Lidocaine is used for dysrhythmias and is not indicated in asystole (AHA, pp. 121-123).

16. **(a)** Many antidepressants have class IA characteristics that prolong QT intervals and may predispose to polymorphic ventricular tachycardia otherwise known as torsades de pointes. Therapy should include a bolus of 2 to 4 g of magnesium sulfate over 5 to 15 minutes (Caruso, p. 210).

17. **(d)** Syncope and chest pain are indications of hypoperfusion. Valve replacement is needed acutely (Massie & Amidon, pp. 350-351).

18. **(b)** Endocarditis may produce subungual splinter hemorrhages and Janeway lesions, which are painless, erythematous lesions of the palms or soles. Osler nodes (painful, violaceous raised lesions on the fingers, toes, or feet) may also be seen. Splenomegaly is an additional helpful sign. Fever in an intravenous drug abuser, especially with a new murmur, is clinically suggestive of endocarditis (Massie & Amidon, p. 354).

19. **(b)** Hypertension is diagnosed after three consecutive BP readings of 140/90 mm Hg or greater. Hypertension should not be diagnosed or treated on the basis of initial readings unless the patient has evidence of acute target organ damage (U.S. Preventive Services Task Force, p. 46).

20. **(a)** Cardiac index and systemic vascular resistance are the most important factors in determining readiness to wean. Intra-aortic balloon pump does not affect pulmonary artery wedge pressure and preload directly. It does affect systemic vascular resistance and coronary artery perfusion pressure (Chulay, Guzzetta, & Dorsey, p. 481).

References

American Heart Association. (1997). *Advanced cardiac life support.* Dallas, TX: American Heart Association.

Baron, R. B. (1998). Nutrition. In L. M. Tierney, Jr., S. J. McPhee, & M. A. Papadakis (Eds.), *Current medical diagnosis and treatment* (37th ed.). Stamford, CT: Appleton & Lange.

Caruso, A. C. (1996). Arrhythmias. In J. Noble (Ed.), *Textbook of primary care medicine* (2nd ed.). St. Louis: Mosby.

Chulay, M., Guzzetta, C., & Dorsey, B. (1997). Advanced cardiovascular concepts. *AACN handbook of critical care nursing.* Stamford, CT: Appleton & Lange.

Dirks, J. (1996). Cardiovascular therapeutic management. In L. D. Urden, M. E. Lough, & K. M. Stacy (Eds.), *Priorities in critical care nursing* (2nd ed.). St. Louis: Mosby.

Ferri, F. (1998). Cardiovascular diseases. *Practical guide to the care of the medical patient* (4th ed.). St. Louis: Mosby.

Kidd, P. S. (1996). Electrocardiographic monitoring and related cardiac interventions. In P. S. Kidd, & K. D. Wagner (Eds.), *High acuity nursing* (2nd ed.). Stamford, CT: Appleton & Lange.

Kimmelstiel, C. D., & Konstam, M. A. (1997). Management of congestive heart failure. In J. Harrington (Ed.), *Consultation in internal medicine* (2nd ed.). St. Louis: Mosby.

Lilly, L. S. (1996). Ischemic heart disease. In J. Noble (Ed.), *Textbook of primary care medicine* (2nd ed.). St. Louis: Mosby.

Massie, B. M. (1998). Systemic hypertension. In L. M. Tierney, Jr., S. J. McPhee, & M. A. Papadakis (Eds.), *Current medical diagnosis and treatment* (37th ed.). Stamford CT: Appleton & Lange.

Massie, B. M., & Amidon, T. A. (1998). Heart. In L. M. Tierney, Jr., S. J. McPhee, & M. A. Papadakis (Eds.), *Current medical diagnosis and treatment* (37th ed.). Stamford CT: Appleton & Lange.

Roberts, S. L. (1996). *Critical care nursing: Assessment and intervention.* Stamford, CT: Appleton & Lange.

Tierney, Jr., L. M., & Messina, L. M. (1998). Blood vessels and lymphatics. In L. M. Tierney, Jr., S. J. McPhee, & M. A. Papadakis (Eds.), *Current medical diagnosis and treatment* (37th ed.). Stamford CT: Appleton & Lange.

U.S. Preventive Services Task Force. (1996). *Guide to clinical preventive services* (2nd ed.). Baltimore: Williams & Wilkins.

Wang, P. J., & Estes, N. A. (1997). Management of atrial fibrillation. In J. Harrington (Ed.), *Consultation in internal medicine* (2nd ed.). St. Louis: Mosby.

Hematological Disorders

Ruth M. Kleinpell

Select one best answer to the following questions.

1. A 57-year-old male presents with a four week history of fatigue. He has no significant past medical history. Vital signs are stable. The Hgb is 11 g/dL, the Hct is 32%, the mean corpuscular volume (MCV) is 75 μ^3, and the mean corpuscular hemoglobin concentration (MCHC) is 30%. These values are most consistent with:

    a. Thalassemia, probably an alpha subtype
    b. A hemodilutional effect
    c. Iron deficiency anemia
    d. A microcytic, normochromic anemia

2. A 48-year-old female presents with a history of pernicious anemia. Pernicious anemia:

    a. Is due to a deficiency of folic acid
    b. Is characterized by late onset neurological symptoms
    c. Is classified as a macrocytic, hypochromic anemia
    d. Is distinguished with a Schilling test

3. A 23-year-old female presents to the emergency room with a history of sickle cell anemia. Which of the following is not accurate with regard to sickle cell crisis?

    a. It frequently presents with shortness of breath and acute pain
    b. Management measures should include platelet transfusion
    c. Sickle cell crises can be precipitated by a recent infection
    d. Narcotic analgesics are often required to relieve crisis pain

4. Chronic lymphocytic leukemia is suspected in a 48-year-old male who has experienced recent fatigue and susceptibility to infections. This type of leukemia:

a. Has a poor prognosis rate in adults as compared to children
b. Has the diagnostic marker of Philadelphia chromosome in most cases
c. Is the most common form of adult leukemia
d. Is known to have a viral etiology

5. Which of the following is characteristic of Non-Hodgkin's lymphoma?

a. It is the most common neoplasm seen in patients aged > 50 years
b. It can be confirmed with Reed-Sternberg cells in lymph node tissue
c. It is classified as an acute lymphocytic leukemia
d. It often presents with painless lymphadenopathy

6. Kate S., a 28-year-old female, was admitted with a three week history of easy bruising and mucosal petechiae. A diagnosis of thrombocytopenia was made after initial laboratory testing revealed a platelet count of 40,000/μL. She reports a sinus infection one week ago, after having the flu for two weeks. She is currently hypotensive at 90/50 mm Hg, febrile at 101.2° F, and appears septic. Although the results of additional laboratory tests are pending the probable diagnosis is:

a. Idiopathic thrombocytopenia purpura (ITP)
b. Possible malignant neoplasm
c. Early disseminated intravascular coagulation (DIC)
d. Acute infectious thrombocytopenia

7. Which of the following statements is accurate with respect to DIC?

a. DIC is confirmed by the presence of elevated fibrin degradation products (FDP) and D-dimer
b. DIC is treated with aminocaproic acid and/or heparin
c. DIC results from increased clotting times and fibrinogen levels
d. DIC is diagnosed by decreasing platelet levels and FDP

8. A 32-year-old female is admitted to the intensive care unit (ICU) with suspected ITP. The ACNP knows that ITP:

a. Results from autoimmune destruction of platelets
b. Results from trauma with profound blood loss
c. Is due to alterations in the coagulation and fibrinolytic systems
d. Occurs due to damaged vascular endothelium

9. A 48-year-old male is admitted to a subacute care facility for aggressive rehabilitation after a motor vehicle accident. He was previously diagnosed with thalassemia. The ACNP caring for this patient has never encountered thalassemia clinically, but remembers from her classes that it:

    a. Is a genetically inherited disorder resulting in abnormal platelet production

    b. Is classified as a macrocytic, hypochromic anemia

    c. Is an autosomal recessive disorder that results in thrombocytopenia

    d. Is a microcytic, hypochromic anemia found in Mediterranean populations

10. Which of the following statements is accurate with regard to folic acid deficiency anemia?

    a. It presents with neurological symptoms

    b. It results from malabsorption of folic acid

    c. It is a macrocytic, normochromic anemia

    d. It is the most common type of anemia

Answers and Rationale

1. **(c)** The laboratory studies reveal a microcytic (MCV < 80 μ^3), hypochromic (MCHC < 32%) anemia. Iron deficiency anemia is the most common form of anemia, and the likely diagnosis for this patient (Wallach, pp. 186-187).

2. **(d)** Pernicious anemia can be distinguished with a Schilling test, which tests the absorption of radiolabeled vitamin B_{12} with and without intrinsic factor administration. Pernicious anemia is due to a lack of intrinsic factor which impairs B_{12} absorption. It is manifested by weakness, fatigue, glossitis and neurological symptoms, including paresthesias, diminished vibratory and position sense, and a positive Romberg and Babinski. Neurological signs and symptoms frequently precede other signs and symptoms of anemia. It is classified as a macrocytic, normochromic anemia (Uphold & Graham, pp. 600-601; Wallach, p. 200).

3. **(b)** Sickle cell crisis is an acute, periodic exacerbation in which the RBC becomes sickle shaped and causes vessel obstruction. Cellular hypoxia results in tissue ischemia which causes pain in the extremities, back, chest, abdomen, and joints. Treatment is directed toward the acute and chronic complications of the disease, and includes oxygen for hypoxemia, antibiotics for infection, fluids for dehydration, analgesics for pain, and occasionally RBC transfusions for anemia (Carey, et al., p. 368; Graber, et al., pp. 207-208).

4. **(c)** Chronic lymphocytic leukemia is the most common form of adult leukemia, found most commonly in persons 50 years of age and older. It is more common in males (Carey, et al., pp. 380-381).

5. **(d)** Non-Hodgkin's lymphoma often presents with painless lymphadenopathy, may have a viral etiology, and is the most common neoplasm for persons aged 20 to 40 years (Carey, et al., p. 380).

6. **(c)** The probable diagnosis given the history, physical findings, and laboratory results is early DIC. DIC varies greatly in clinical severity and may present with either bleeding or thrombosis. Patients presenting with early DIC demonstrate disturbance in hemostasis with easy bruising and petechia on mucosal membranes. Thrombocytopenia (platelets < 150,000 /μL), hypofibrinogenemia (fibrinogen < 170 mg/dL), decreased RBC, increased fibrin

degredation products (FDP > 45 μg/dL or present at > 1:100 dilution), prolonged PT (> 19 seconds) and PTT (> 42 seconds) are also seen. Although thrombocytopenia is found in ITP, the patient's clinical findings are suggestive of a concurrent infectious process and possible sepsis, conditions which precipitate DIC. Malignant neoplasms do not characteristically present with thrombocytopenia (Marino, pp. 712-713; Wallach, pp. 246-247).

7. **(a)** Elevated FDP and D-dimer give a predictive accuracy of 96% for diagnosing DIC. DIC results from increased clotting times and decreased fibrinogen levels. Decreased platelet levels and increased FDP are seen (Wallach, pp. 246-247).

8. **(a)** Idiopathic thrombocytopenia purpura (ITP) is an acquired thrombocytopenia resulting from autoimmune destruction of platelets with or without suppression of thrombopoiesis. ITP can occur acutely and may present with an abrupt decrease in platelets and bleeding, or can occur as a chronic disorder, causing mild to severe thrombocytopenia. ITP occurs in women aged 20 to 40 as compared to men by a ratio of 3:1 (Grodzin, et al., pp. 416-417).

9. **(d)** Thalessemia is a genetically inherited disorder resulting in abnormal hemoglobin production and hypochromic, microcytic anemia, found in Mediterranean populations (Carey, et al., pp. 362-363).

10. **(c)** Folic acid deficiency anemia is a macrocytic, normochromic anemia due to folic acid deficiency which is caused by inadequate intake or malabsorption of folic acid. Symptoms include fatigue, dyspnea on exertion, pallor, headache, anorexia, and glossitis. Folic acid deficiency anemia is differentiated from pernicious anemia by neurologic symptoms, such as paresthesias and loss of vibratory sense, which are present only in pernicious anemia (Carey, et al., pp. 364-366; Uphold & Graham, pp. 599-601).

References

Carey, C., Lee, H., & Woeltje, K. (1998). *The Washington manual of medical therapeutics.* Philadelphia: Lippincott-Raven.

Graber, M., Toth, P., & Herting, R. (1997). *The family practice handbook.* St. Louis: Mosby.

Grodzin, C., Schwartz, S., & Bone, R. (1996). *Diagnostic strategies for internal medicine.* St. Louis: Mosby.

Marino, P. (1998). *The ICU book* (2nd ed.). Baltimore: Williams & Wilkins.

Uphold, C., & Graham, M. (1994). *Clinical guidelines in adult health.* Gainesville, Florida: Barmarrae Books.

Wallach, J. (1998). *Handbook of interpretation of diagnostic tests.* Philadelphia: Lippincott-Raven.

Immunological Disorders

Ruth M. Kleinpell

Select one best answer to the following questions.

1. A 21-year-old male was diagnosed with HIV one year ago. The management of his HIV infection includes $CD4^+$ count testing:

   a. Every 6 months when the $CD4^+$ count is > 600 cells/μL
   b. Every 3 months when the $CD4^+$ count is > 500 cells/μL
   c. Every 6 months when the $CD4^+$ count is between 200 and 600 cells/μL
   d. Every 3 months when the $CD4^+$ count is < 800 cells/μL

2. Your patient was diagnosed with HIV. This is his first visit for general health evaluation, counseling, and discussion of treatment. His absolute $CD4^+$ count is 500 cells/μL and viral load is 25,000 copies/mL. With regard to antiretroviral treatment, you tell the patient that based on his laboratory tests:

   a. Antiretroviral treatment is not appropriate at this time
   b. The two medicines that he will start with are called zidovudine and zalcitabine
   c. The two medicines that he will start with are called ritonavir and lamivudine
   d. The two medicines that he will start with are called nelfinavir and delavirdine

3. A 72-year-old female presents to the outpatient clinic with complaints of joint stiffness and Heberden's nodes. These are characteristic findings associated with which of the following conditions?

   a. Rheumatoid arthritis
   b. Gout
   c. Osteoarthritis
   d. Osteoporosis

4. Rheumatoid arthritis is suspected in a 54-year-old female who has a one year

history of weakness. Which of the following statements is not true regarding rheumatoid arthritis?

   a. Rheumatoid arthritis is a chronic inflammatory disease of the synovial joint and tendon sheath

   b. Baker's cysts, or synovial cysts of the popliteal space, are common

   c. Morning stiffness and joint pain are characteristic symptoms

   d. It results in joint degeneration which causes deterioration of bone formation at the joint surfaces

5. Mr R., a 65-year-old male, presented to the outpatient clinic with a history of a malar discoid rash, photosensitivity, and oral ulcers. Laboratory testing reveals a positive rheumatoid factor and positive antinuclear antibody test. The most likely diagnosis is:

   a. Rheumatoid arthritis

   b. Osteomyelitis

   c. Systemic lupus erythematosus

   d. Mixed connective tissue disease

6. Which of the following are not associated with immunosuppression?

   a. Malnutrition

   b. Age

   c. WBC proliferation

   d. Malignancy

7. Mr. B., a 27-year-old male who is HIV positive, presents to the urgent care center with a history of cough, fever, malaise, and fatigue for the past week. He was relatively healthy prior to this and a purified protein derivative (PPD) test six months ago was negative. He was recently started on antiretroviral therapy for a decreasing $CD4^+$ count. The most likely diagnosis is:

   a. Adverse drug reaction

   b. An opportunistic infection

   c. Sepsis

   d. Antiretroviral drug resistance

8. Ms R., a 21-year-old female, presents with a persistent cough and upper respiratory symptoms for two weeks. She has a history of recurrent pneumonia and was treated three times between the ages of 12 and 14, twice as an inpatient.

Her medical history is significant for asthma and rhinitis. Which of the following is the least significant aspect of the history when assessing an immunodeficiency?

   a. History of infections
   b. Vaccination history
   c. Family history
   d. Current medications

9. Mr. H. is a 48-year-old male who presents to the emergency room with difficulty breathing. He reports that he experienced a tingling sensation in his lips and began coughing about one hour ago, which progressed to wheezing. He has no significant past medical history. Further questioning reveals that he had been attending a wedding reception at a nearby hotel where the groom and bridal party were smoking cigars. The most likely diagnosis is:

   a. Asthma attack
   b. Early pneumonia
   c. Acute bronchitis
   d. An allergic reaction

10. A 66-year-old female with a history of joint pain is being evaluated for osteoarthritis. Which of the following is not associated with osteoarthritis?

   a. Obesity
   b. Trauma
   c. Previous fracture
   d. Demineralization of bone

Answers and Rationale

1. **(a)** CD4$^+$ count testing should be measured once every six months when the CD4$^+$ count is > 600 cells/μL and at least every three months when the CD4$^+$ count is between 200 cells/μL and 600 cells/μL. More frequent measurements may be desirable if there is evidence of rapid decline in cell count or if the patient's symptoms become more severe (Carey, et al., pp. 288-290).

2. **(b)** Patients never before treated for HIV are given first line treatment which consists of two nucleoside analogs. Protease inhibitors and nonnucleoside reverse transcriptase inhibitors are not considered first line treatment (Katz & Hollander, pp. 1222-1224).

3. **(c)** Heberden's nodes (enlargement of the distal interphalangeal joints) are seen in osteoarthritis. (Carey, et al., pp. 257-258; Uphold & Graham, pp. 540-543).

4. **(d)** Rheumatoid arthritis is a chronic inflammatory disease of the synovial joint and tendon sheath. The proximal interphalangeal and metacarpophalangeal joints are often affected. Morning stiffness, which lasts several hours, and joint pain or stiffness are common symptoms. Baker's cysts, or synovial cysts of the popliteal space, are common in patients with rheumatoid arthritis (Carey, et al., pp. 252-253; Uphold & Graham, pp. 546-549).

5. **(c)** While a positive test for rheumatoid factor is seen in chronic inflammatory and autoimmune diseases including subacute bacterial endocarditis, osteomyelitis, granulomatous infections or diseases, rheumatoid arthritis, systemic lupus erythematosus (SLE), Sjogren's syndrome and mixed connective tissue disease, a positive antinuclear antibody is seen in the majority of patients with SLE. The symptoms manifested by the patient, in conjunction with the laboratory tests, indicate a diagnosis of SLE (Carey, et al., p. 471; Grodzin, et al., p. 761).

6. **(c)** Immunosupression can result from a variety of factors including chronic systemic illness, malignancy, solid organ or bone marrow transplantation, and congenital and acquired conditions. Other factors such as age, malnutrition, uremia, alcoholism, and steroid therapy can also result in immunosuppression. Malnutrition impairs the cellular functioning of T cells, and with

age atrophy of the thymus gland results in lower levels of circulating T cells (Graber, et al., p. 682).

7. **(b)** The patient is most likely experiencing a pulmonary opportunistic infection. Although he had been healthy, a decreasing $CD4^+$ count would put the patient at increased risk for an opportunistic infection. Antiretroviral drug resistance is most commonly manifested with anemia, nausea, neutropenia, and/or neuropathy (Carey, et al., pp. 289-292).

8. **(b)** A patient presenting with frequent infections should have a thorough history of all known infections since childhood. Specific pathogens should be documented if known. Family history is an essential factor in diagnosing genetically transmitted disorders. Current medications are also important information as medications such as phenytoin have been known to cause an IgA deficiency that is reversible (Grodzin, et al., pp. 12-14).

9. **(d)** The most likely diagnosis is an allergy attack. The symptoms of tingling sensation, coughing, wheezing and difficulty breathing indicate an allergic response, possibly related to a food, drink, or smoke allergen (Carey, et al., pp. 215-216).

10. **(d)** Osteoarthritis is a disorder of the joint which causes deterioration of articular joint surfaces. Osteoarthritis can occur without obvious cause, and is also associated with obesity, family history, and trauma (Uphold & Graham, pp. 540-543).

References

Carey, C., Lee, H., & Woeltje, K. (1998). *The Washington manual of medical therapeutics.* Philadelphia: Lippincott-Raven.

Graber, M., Toth, P., & Herting, R. (1997). *The family practice handbook.* St. Louis: Mosby.

Grodzin, C., Schwartz, S., & Bone, R. (1996). *Diagnostic strategies for internal medicine.* St. Louis: Mosby.

Katz, M. H., & Hollander, H. (1998). HIV infection. In L. M. Tierney, Jr., S. J. McPhee, & M. A. Papadakis (Eds.). *Current medical diagnosis and treatment* (37th ed.). pp. 1204-1230). Stamford, CT: Appleton & Lange.

Uphold, C., & Graham, M. (1994). *Clinical guidelines in adult health.* Gainesville, FL: Barmarrae Books.

Endocrine Disorders

Candis Morrison

Select one best answer to the following questions.

1. A 30-year-old patient with a history of type 2 diabetes is brought into the emergency department (ED) in a near comatose state. His heart rate is 124 bpm and BP is 90/50 mm Hg. Initial laboratory evaluation reveals a blood glucose level of 625 g/dL, with negative serum ketones. Urine glucose is 4+ and ketones are present in the urine. Serum potassium is 4.0 mEq/dL and serum osmolality is 320 mOsm/L. Which feature distinguishes diabetic ketoacidosis from hyperosmolar hyperglycemic nonketotic coma in this patient?

   a. Hyperglycemia
   b. Elevated serum osmolality
   c. Normal serum potassium
   d. Negative serum ketones

2. The primary concern in the management of a patient with acute diabetic ketoacidosis or hyperosmolar coma is:

   a. Potentiation of insulin utilization
   b. Normalization of glucose levels
   c. Correction of potassium and chloride
   d. The replacement of salt and water deficits

3. J. M. is a 19-year-old patient with type 1 diabetes. He administered his NPH insulin at 8 a.m. During midmorning he developed nausea and vomited two times, therefore missing lunch. Upon physical examination he is alert and oriented, but appears anxious. He is slightly diaphoretic, his heart rate is 108 bpm and he is breathing 20 times per minute. Your initial treatment for this patient consists of:

   a. 0.5 mg glucagon IM
   b. 100 cc of D_5W IV

    c. 25 mL of $D_{50}W$ IV

    d. 4 oz orange juice p.o.

4. The ACNP has been managing a patient with type 1 diabetes for several months. He was formerly controlled on split dose insulin and self glucose monitoring. Since his vision has deteriorated, he is unable to use his self monitoring equipment. Which laboratory test would be the most unbiased means of determining glycemic control in this patient?

    a. 2 hour post-prandial serum glucose
    b. Fasting serum glucose
    c. 24 hour urine glucose/ketone assay
    d. Hemoglobin A_{1c}

5. R.J. is a 37-year-old secretary presenting to urgent care with symptoms of severe headache, intermittent palpitations, nausea, vomiting, nervousness, irritability, and dyspnea. Symptoms began abruptly this morning. Her occupational health nurse reports that her BP was 200/110 mm Hg when taken in the clinic before referral. Current medication includes Premarin 0.625 mg q.d. status post total hysterectomy and bilateral oophorectomy two years ago. Past medical history is noncontributory. Objective findings reveal: Temp 37.8° C, BP 160/90 mm Hg sitting and 130/70 mm Hg standing, heart rate 104 bpm sitting and 128 bpm standing, and resp 24 bpm. Skin is warm and moist. Her chest is clear to auscultation. Cardiovascular examination reveals a regular but rapid rate and a grade II systolic murmur heard best over the precordium. Neurological examination is unremarkable with the exception of a sustained tremor bilaterally. To differentiate between two possible causes of this symptom complex, which two tests would be most helpful?

    a. Dexamethasone suppression test and an MRI of the brain
    b. Adrenocorticotropic hormone (ACTH) stimulation test and chest CT scan
    c. Glucose tolerance test and erythrocyte sedimentation rate
    d. Thyroid function studies and urinary catecholamines

6. The ACNP is evaluating a patient who has been maintained on long term prednisone therapy for treatment of asthma. Typical signs of cortisol excess are noted—central obesity, ecchymosis, and purple striae. Iatrogenic Cushing's syndrome is associated with the adverse metabolic effects of:

    a. Hypoglycemia
    b. Osteoporosis
    c. Diabetes insipidus
    d. Hyperkalemia

7. A 49-year-old male complains of intermittent episodes of severe headache and diaphoresis. He reports that his heart often races and he gets dizzy spells. He has lost 10 pounds over the past 2 to 3 months. Upon examination he demonstrates marked orthostatic hypotension. Ophthalmoscopic examination reveals arterial narrowing. Cardiac auscultation reveals an S_4 sound. ECG reveals left ventricular hypertrophy (LVH). Serum multichemical analysis (SMA) 20, thyroid function tests, and CBC with differential are all within normal limits. You strongly suspect:

    a. Adrenal insufficiency
    b. Renal artery stenosis
    c. Thyroid storm
    d. Pheochromocytoma

8. The most sensitive and specific test for supected pheochromocytoma is:

    a. 24 hour urine metanephrines
    b. Serum catecholamines
    c. 24 hour urine catecholamines
    d. Serum vanillylmandelic acid

9. A 33-year-old obese white female returns for her third BP check for a diagnosis of hypertension. On further questioning she complains of polyuria, polyphagia, weight gain, amenorrhea and easy bruisability. Physical examination reveals truncal obesity, mild hirsutism and bilateral peripheral edema. Laboratory examination reveals a random glucose of 285 mg/dL. You suspect:

    a. Diabetes mellitus
    b. Diabetes insipidus
    c. Cushing's disease
    d. Hypothyroidism

10. You are examining a 42-year-old female who claims to have been obese since childhood. She insists that she complies with a prescribed 1500 calorie diet and has tried multiple diets and exercise plans to lose weight. She also complains of cold intolerance, fatigue, constipation and menorrhagia. Upon physical examination she has course, dry skin, her voice is somewhat hoarse, and her deep tendon reflexes demonstrate delayed response. Which test would be the most appropriate to begin her evaluation?

    a. 24 hour urine metanephrines
    b. Thyroid stimulating hormone (TSH)

    c. T_3 and T_4

    d. Thyroglobulins

11. Your insulin dependent patient is on split doses of NPH. His morning self glucose monitoring has consistently revealed elevated morning readings. You order a 3 a.m. glucose which is also elevated. This implies:

    a. Dawn phenomenon

    b. Smogyi phenomenon

    c. Insulin allergy

    d. Reactive hypoglycemia

12. A 46-year-old woman presents with symptoms of increased sweating, intolerance of heat, increased appetite, and a weight loss of 10 pounds in the preceding three weeks. She has been unable to sleep at night and has become irritable. She has missed her last two periods and believes that her symptoms are menopausal. Upon examination her heart rate is rapid at 112 bpm. Her skin is warm and moist. Examination of her neck reveals a diffuse goiter. She has a fine hand tremor. Initial laboratory values reveal a mild normochromic, normocytic anemia, an increased erythrocyte sedimentation rate, and suppressed serum TSH. This clincial picture is highly suggestive of:

    a. Autoimmune hemolytic anemia

    b. Menopause

    c. Thyrotoxicosis

    d. Pheochromocytoma

13. A. S. is a 32-year-old patient complaining of headache and diplopia of recent onset. Review of systems reveals a four year history of irregular menses and a bilateral milky nipple discharge that is spontaneous. Family history is negative for breast and gynecological cancers. An important screening test for this patient would be serum:

    a. Prolactin

    b. Metanephrines

    c. Estradiol

    d. Cortisol

14. While performing an admission history and physical examination on a patient scheduled for an elective cholecystectomy, you detect a 1 cm firm, nontender thyroid nodule. The patient is completely asymptomatic. Thyroid function tests are within normal limits. Which of the following is the best modality to assess this nodule for malignancy?

a. Thyroid ultrasound
b. CT scan
c. Fine needle aspiration
d. Serum thyroid antibodies

15. Acute adrenocortical insufficiency is a medical emergency. If suspected, one should administer:

a. $D_{50}W$ and hypotonic saline
b. Glucagon and potassium chloride
c. Epinephrine and D_5W
d. Hydrocortisone and saline

Answers and Rationale

1. **(d)** Both conditions present with hyperglycemia, (hyperosmolar, hyperglycemic nonketotic (HHNK) coma often with a more dramatic glucose elevation). Both also demonstrate hyperosmolality and can have normal potassium early in the course. Eventually potassium is depleted (Nelson, pp. 268-269).

2. **(d)** The primary concern is replacement of salt and water deficits. Patients with acute diabetic ketoacidosis present with hypovolemia, and incipient, or overt, shock. The paramount concern is the replacement of salt and water deficits. Glucose and electrolyte abnormalities will be less problematic as salt and water deficits are normalized (Daly, pp. 571-572).

3. **(d)** This patient is exhibiting signs and symptoms of hypoglycemia. Treatment for hypoglycemia is 10 to 15 grams of carbohydrate. Candy or fruit juice should be administered to an alert patient. If the patient were unable to take p.o. nutrition, the only choice providing this amount is the $D_{50}W$ (Daly, pp. 571-572).

4. **(d)** Hemoglobin A_{1c} assay can serve as an unbiased means of determining glycemic control and for patients without, or unable to use, home blood glucose meters, these tests are far more accurate determinants of glycemic control than office drawn fasting or random blood glucose. The percentage of glycosylated hemoglobin is highly correlated with mean blood glucose values for the preceding two months and thus serves as an accurate benchmark of overall glycemic control (Chipkin, et al., pp. 483-484).

5. **(d)** This picture is most consistent with the diagnosis of pheochromocytoma or thyrotoxicosis. With a clinical picture of hypermetabolism, normal thyroid functions (T_4, FT_4, T_3, and TSH) would eliminate the possibility of a thyroid hormone excess, supporting the diagnosis of pheochromocytoma (Fitzgerald, pp. 1080-1082).

6. **(b)** Osteoporosis occurs in up to 50% of patients treated with chronic glucocorticoids. Hyperglycemia and hypokalemia are potential electrolyte derangements (Brunt & Melby, pp. 522-523).

7. **(d)** These signs and symptoms are consistent with pheochromocytoma. The manifestations of pheochromocytoma are varied. It typically causes attacks with severe headache, palpitations, tachycardia, profuse sweating, vasomotor changes, precordial or abdominal pain, increasing nervousness and irritability, increased appetite, and loss of weight. Physical findings may include hypertension, either in attacks or sustained, and often severe. Patients may show cardiac enlargement, postural tachycardia and hypotension (Wang & Cooper, pp. 290-292).

8. **(a)** Metanephrine measurement is the most sensitive and specific test, because foods and medication have less effect on its levels. Beta adrenergic blocking drugs and radio contrast dyes can alter catecholamine metabolites in an acidified 24 hour urine collection (Wang & Cooper, pp. 290-292).

9. **(c)** Cushing's disease presents with symptoms of amenorrhea, polydipsia, polyuria, and signs of hypertension, acne, central obesity, and impaired glucose tolerance (Fitzgerald, pp. 1075-1076).

10. **(b)** This clinical picture is consistent with hypothyroidsim. TSH is increased with primary hypothyroidism and is the appropriate screening test (Fitzgerald, 1049-1051).

11. **(a)** To differentiate between Dawn and Smogyi phenomenon (two causes of a.m. hyperglycemia) a 3 a.m. glucose is ordered. When it is high, this implies nocturnal insensitivity to insulin. This is known as the Dawn phenomenon. If the 3 a.m. glucose was low, you would label it Smogyi effect (Karam, p. 1118).

12. **(c)** Thyrotoxicosis is differentiated from other causes of hypermetabolism by TSH assay. It is the best test for thyrotoxicosis and is suppressd in the majority of cases. Serum T_3, T_4, thyroid resin uptake, and free thyroxine are all usually increased (Fitzgerald, pp. 1051-1053).

13. **(a)** The major concern in this case is a prolactin secreting macroadenoma. If this were the cause of the symptoms, serum prolactin would be elevated in excess of 250 ng/mL. This should prompt MRI evaluation and neurosurgical referral (Wand, pp. 274-275).

14. **(c)** Fine needle aspiration/biopsy is the best way to assess a nodule for malignancy. This test has supplanted thyroid scanning as it provides actual tissue for a pathological analysis (Fitzgerald, p. 1058).

15. (d) Acute adrenal insufficiency is an emergency due to acute insufficiency of cortisol. If suspected, it is important to draw a serum cortisol but to initiate therapy with 100 to 300 mg of hydrocortisone immediately and infuse salt to help correct the profound dehydration that results from this condition (Fitzgerald, pp. 1072-1073).

References

Brunt, M. J., & Melby, J. C. (1996). Adrenal gland disorders. In J. Noble (Ed.), *Textbook of primary care medicine* (2nd ed.). St. Louis: Mosby.

Chipkin, S. R., Gottlieb, P. A., Bogorad, D. D., & Parker, F. (1997). Diabetes mellitus. In J. Noble (Ed.), *Textbook of primary care medicine* (2nd ed.). St. Louis: Mosby.

Daly, J., & Harrington, J. T. (1997). Diabetes. In J. Harrington (Ed.), *Consultation in internal medicine* (2nd ed.). St. Louis: Mosby.

Fitzgerald, P. A. (1998). Endocrinology. In L. M Tierney, Jr., S. J. McPhee, & M. A. Papadakis (Eds.), *Current medical diagnosis and treatment* (37th ed.). Stamford CT: Appleton & Lange.

Karam, J. H. (1998). Diabetes mellitus and hypoglycemia. In L. M. Tierney, Jr., S. J. McPhee, & M. A. Papadakis (Eds.), *Current medical diagnosis and treatment* (37th ed.). Stamford CT: Appleton & Lange.

Nelson, S. J. (1996). Disorders of glucose circulation and uptake. In H. L. Greene (Ed.), *Clinical medicine* (2nd ed.). St. Louis: Mosby.

Wand, G. S., & Cooper, D. S. (1996). Adrenal disorders. In J. D. Stobo, D. B. Hellmann, P. W. Ladenson, B. G. Petty, & T. A. Traill (Eds.), *The principles and practice of medicine* (23rd ed.). Stamford, CT: Appleton & Lange.

Wang, G. S. (1997). Pituitary disorders. In J. D. Stobo, D. B. Hellmann, P. W. Ladenson, B. G. Petty, & T. A. Traill (Eds.), *The principles and practice of medicine* (23rd ed.). Stamford, CT: Appleton & Lange.

Gastrointestinal Disorders

Ruth M. Kleinpell

Select one best answer to the following questions.

1. Ms. R., a 47-year-old female, presents with a four week history of dyspepsia. Which of the following should not be included in assessing important historical information?

   a. Use of aspirin or nonsteroidal anti-inflammatory drugs (NSAID)
   b. Stress
   c. Alcohol and cigarette use
   d. Dietary protein intake

2. Mr. B. is a 32-year-old male who presents with complaints of vague epigastric discomfort and heartburn for the past month. He relates that his mother had ulcers and he thinks that he has one. The epigastric discomfort usually begins two hours after eating and he finds that food helps to relieve the pain. The most likely diagnosis is:

   a. Gastric ulcer
   b. Gastritis
   c. Duodenal ulcer
   d. Gastroesophageal reflux disease

3. A 52-year-old male presents to the emergency room with epigastric pain. Upon diagnostic evaluation, he is found to be anemic. Epigastric pain and anemia are commonly found in patients with:

   a. Peptic ulcer disease
   b. Gastritis
   d. Gastroesophageal reflux disease
   e. Gastrointestinal virus

4. Mr. J. is a 32-year-old male who presents with a four day history of fever, left

lower abdominal pain and tenderness, and diarrhea. He denies any history of colon problems. The most likely diagnosis is:

    a. Crohn's disease
    b. Diverticulitis
    c. Ulcerative colitis
    d. Ischemic colitis

5. The ACNP is assessing a patient to rule out appendicitis. During the examination the patient is found to have right lower quadrant pain. This is known as:

    a. McBurney's sign
    b. The obturator sign
    c. The psoas sign
    d. Murphy's sign

6. Peritonitis is suspected in a 66-year-old female in the emergency room. Which of the following are not abdominal manifestations of peritonitis?

    a. Pain
    b. Distention
    c. Rigidity
    d. Rebound pain

Questions 7 and 8 refer to the following scenario.

Ms. P. is a 45-year-old female who presents with jaundice and a three week history of anorexia, malaise, and intermittent right upper quadrant pain. Her initial laboratory values reveal an aspartate aminotransferase (AST) of 1250 mg/dL, alanine aminotransferase (ALT) of 985 mg/dL, total bilirubin of 2.2 mg/dL, and alkaline phosphatase of 158 mg/dL.

7. Which of the following would not be an appropriate differential diagnosis?

    a. Viral hepatitis
    b. Hepatic encephalopathy
    c. Drug hepatotoxicity
    d. Hepatic neoplasm

8. Additional laboratory values revealed antihepatitis A virus (anti-HAV) (IgM) negative, hepatits B surface antigen (HBsAg) positive, hepatitis B core antibody (anti-HBc) (IgM) positive, anti-hepatitis B core antigen (HBeAg) positive,

antibody hepatitis C virus (anti-HCV) negative, and HIV negative. What is the correct interpretation of the serology tests?

    a. The patient has acute hepatitis C

    b. The patient has acute hepatitis B

    c. The patient does not have active disease but was exposed to hepatitis B previously

    d. The patient has acute hepatitis A

9. A 34-year-old traveling salesman recently returning from Mexico was admitted to the stepdown unit with suspected viral hepatitis. He has no risk factors for parenteral hepatitis. Given his travel history, the ACNP knows he is at highest risk for:

    a. Hepatitis A

    b. Hepatitis B

    c. Hepatitis C

    d. Hepatitis D

10. Acute pancreatitis is suspected in a 54-year-old female in the ICU. Which of the following is not typically found in acute pancreatitis?

    a. Elevated serum amylase

    b. Epigastric to left upper quadrant pain

    c. Positive Murphy's sign

    d. Abdominal distention, nausea and vomiting

11. A 42-year-old male presents to the clinic with bloody diarrhea. Bloody diarrhea is a hallmark symptom of:

    a. Ulcerative colitis

    b. Crohn's disease

    c. Diverticulitis

    d. Bowel infarction

12. Bowel obstruction can vary in its presentation depending upon the patient's general state of health, location of the obstruction, and time since onset. Which of the following physical findings is not seen in any typical bowel obstruction scenario?

    a. Cramping abdominal pain

    b. Abdominal distention

    c. High pitched, tinkling bowel sounds

    d. Rebound tenderness

13. In the emergency room a 32-year-old male is found to have a psoas sign. The psoas sign is found in patients with:

    a. Cholecystitis
    b. Appendicitis
    c. Peritonitis
    d. Acute diverticulitis

14. Mr. S., a 49-year-old male, is brought to the emergency room by his roommate who relates that the patient has been vomiting bright red blood for two days. He has a history of alcohol abuse. Current vital signs are as follows: Temp 99.2° F, heart rate 110 bpm (sinus tachycardia), blood pressure 90/60 mm Hg, resp 32 bpm. He is alert but lethargic and denies current abdominal pain. Which of the following is not indicated in the initial management of this patient?

    a. Immediate IV access
    b. Laboratory screening, type and crossmatch
    c. Endoscopy
    d. Crystalloid infusion

15. Health care providers are becoming much more conservative with respect to ordering transfusions of blood products. However, there are times when an immediate transfusion is indicated. Which of the following is an absolute indication for transfusion?

    a. Continued bleeding
    b. Low hemoglobin and hematocrit
    c. Vital signs remaining unstable despite crystalloid infusions
    d. Platelet count < 10,000/μL

16. Which of the following statements about upper gastrointestinal (UGI) tract hemorrhage is accurate?

    a. Most acute UGI bleeding stops spontaneously without intervention
    b. Surgical intervention or endoscopy is often needed
    c. UGI bleeding has stopped when no further bloody vomiting occurs
    d. UGI bleeding has stopped when the hematocrit is stable for 24 hours

17. Esophageal varices is a common etiology of upper gastrointestinal bleeding. Which of the following is not indicated in the initial management of esophageal varices?

    a. Sclerotherapy or banding

    b. Vasopressin

    c. Balloon tamponade for controlled bleeding

    d. Surgical shunting

18. Agitation, asterixis, and fetor hepaticus are clinical findings consistent with:

    a. Renal failure

    b. Hcpatitis

    c. Nephrotic syndrome

    d. Cirrhosis

19. A routine pre-employment physical examination of a 48-year-old male reveals a guaiac positive stool upon digital rectal examination. The ACNP knows that this finding should be followed-up with:

    a. Colonoscopy

    b. Air contrast barium enema

    c. Repeat testing

    d. Flexible sigmoidoscopy

20. Mrs. R. was admitted to the general medical service last week for intravenous antibiotic management of an infected diabetic ulcer. Today she has developed frequent, watery diarrhea. The ACNP orders a stool specimen for:

    a. Ova and parasites

    b. Occult blood

    c. *Clostridium difficile*

    d. *Eschericia coli*

Answers and Rationale

1. **(d)** Dyspepsia often occurs with peptic ulcer disease, and the history should assess risk factors for peptic ulcer disease. Aspirin or NSAID interfere with the normal mucosal defense mechanisms and may cause a topical irritation that directly damages the mucosa. Other risk factors include psychological stress, alcohol consumption, caffeine use, and cigarette smoking. Smokers have an increased incidence of ulcer recurrence as well as impaired healing (Graber, et al., pp. 169-172).

2. **(c)** The most likely diagnosis is duodenal ulcer. Duodenal ulcers comprise 80% of all peptic ulcers, have a higher incidence in males and have a familial disposition. The epigastric pain is often relieved by food or antacids (Uphold & Graham, pp. 412-415).

3. **(a)** Epigastric pain with anemia is commonly found with a diagnosis of peptic ulcer disease (Uphold & Graham, pp. 412-415).

4. **(c)** Diverticulitis is characterized by fever and lower abdominal pain and tenderness. Hemoccult positive stools can occur in 25% of cases (Grodzin, et al., p. 291).

5. **(a)** McBurney's sign is right lower abdominal pain $\frac{1}{3}$ the distance from the iliac crest to the umbilicus and is characterisitic of appendicitis (Mladenovic, p. 163).

6. **(d)** Clinical manifestations of peritonitis include abdominal pain, distention, and rigidity. Anorexia, nausea and vomiting, fever, and chills can also be present (Parsons & Wiener-Kronish, p. 269).

7. **(b)** Suspected differential diagnoses include hepatitis, drug hepatotoxicity and hepatic neoplasm. Although hemochromatosis can present with elevation of transaminases, it is an autosomal recessive iron storage disorder usually presenting in the fifth or sixth decade in men (Grodzin, et al., pp. 245-247).

8. **(b)** The patient has acute hepatitis B. Since the HBeAg is also positive, he is considered highly infectious. Acute hepatitis B can be distinguished from

chronic hepatitis B by the presence of IgM anti-HBc antibody at the onset of disease. HBeAg is positive during the period of high infectivity and reflects viral replication (Grodzin, et al., p. 249).

9. **(a)** Fecal-oral transmission of viral hepatitis is seen in hepatitis A, E and G viruses (Grodzin, et al., p. 247).

10. **(c)** Findings in acute pancreatitis include elevated serum amylase and epigastric to left upper quadrant pain which is knifelike or boring in quality. Abdominal distention, nausea, and vomiting are frequent findings. Murphy's sign, extreme tenderness to subhepatic area with palpation during deep inspiration, is seen in cholecystitis (Graber, et al., pp. 176-178).

11. **(a)** Bloody diarrhea is a hallmark symptom of ulcerative colitis (Carey, et al., p. 317).

12. **(d)** Physical findings in bowel obstruction include cramping abdominal pain, abdominal distention and high pitched, tinkling bowel sounds (Graber, et al., pp. 407-409).

13. **(b)** The psoas sign (right or left lower quadrant pain with passive extension of the right leg at the hip when the patient is lying on the left side) results from psoas muscle irritation, and is positive with acute appendicitis (Mladenovic, p. 162).

14. **(c)** Initial steps in management of GI bleeding include obtaining IV access, laboratory screening, and type and crossmatch. Patients with hemodynamic compromise should be given immediate volume replacement. Endoscopy would not be an initial treatment but would be indicated for continued bleeding (Parsons & Wiener-Kronish, pp. 253-257).

15. **(c)** Blood transfusion for GI bleeding is indicated if vital signs remain unstable despite crystalloid infusion. Continued bleeding may not necessitate transfusions if blood loss is not significant. Blood transfusions may not be given for low hemoglobin or hematocrit levels until hematocrits fall below the 27 to 30% range (Carey, et al., pp. 302-303).

16. **(a)** Approximately 85% of all acute UGI bleeding stops spontaneously. Frequent gastric aspirate that remains free of blood is the best early sign of cessation (Carey, et al., pp. 302-308).

17. **(d)** Initial treatment for esophageal varices include sclerotherapy or banding, pharmacologic therapy with vasopressin, and balloon tamponade with a Sengstaken-Blakemore tube to control hemorrhage. Shunting is reserved for variceal bleeding that is refractory to other measures, and is associated with 25% to 50% mortality (Grodin, et al., pp. 254-255).

18. **(d)** Clinical findings seen with cirrhosis include agitation, asterixis (a flapping motion seen when the patient is asked to hold his arms horizontally with hands extended at the wrists), and fetor hepaticus, a feculent-fruity odor of the breath (Grodzin, et al., p. 257).

19. **(c)** Guaiac positive stool obtained from a digital rectal examination requires repeat testing (Carey, et al., p. 309).

20. **(c)** *Clostridium difficile* diarrhea can occur after beginning antibiotic therapy, usually 4 to 9 days after initiation, but symptoms can occur up to 6 weeks after antibiotics are discontinued (Marino, pp. 534-537).

References

Carey, C., Lee, H., & Woeltje, K. (1998). *The Washington manual of medical therapeutics.* Philadelphia: Lippincott-Raven.

Graber, M., Toth, P., & Herting, R. (1997). *The family practice handbook.* St. Louis: Mosby.

Grodzin, C., Schwartz, S., & Bone, R. (1996). *Diagnostic strategies for internal medicine.* St. Louis: Mosby.

Marino, P. (1998). *The ICU book* (2nd ed.). Baltimore: Williams & Wilkins.

Mladenovic, J. (1995). *Primary care secrets.* St. Louis: Mosby.

Parsons, P., & Wiener-Kronish, J. (1998). *Critical care secrets.* St. Louis: Mosby.

Uphold, C., & Graham, M. (1994). *Clinical guidelines in adult health.* Gainesville, Florida: Barmarrae Books.

Renal/Genitourinary
Disorders, STDs

Ruth M. Kleinpell

Select one best answer to the following questions.

Questions 1 and 2 refer to the following scenario.

Mary P., an 18-year-old female, presents to the ED with a three day history of dysuria and low back pain. She denies any previous episodes. A urinalysis reveals > 10 WBC/HPF. Urine leukocyte esterase and nitrites are positive. She is currently febrile at 100.8° F and reports having chills last evening.

1. The most likely diagnosis is:

    a. Cystitis
    b. Gonorrhea
    c. Pyelonephritis
    d. Renal abscess

2. The indicated treatment for Mary P. is:

    a. Hospitalization for intravenous (IV) antibiotics until afebrile
    b. Management on an outpatient basis with a 14 day course of antibiotics
    c. Hospitalization if pregnant and nausea/vomiting is present
    d. Management on an outpatient basis with three days of antibiotic therapy

3. The ACNP is called to see a patient on an inpatient stepdown unit for oliguria. The patient underwent a transurethral resection of the prostate (TURP) two days ago. The nurse reports that the urine was straw colored without clots during the previous shift. There is no return from a 100 cc sterile foley irrigation. The patient is alert and reports no discomfort. The operative report indicates the patient had an episode of intraoperative hypotension but vital signs have

been stable since. How would the ACNP best differentiate prerenal vs. intrarenal oliguria?

a. Administer a fluid bolus of 500 cc 0.9% NSS and monitor the response
b. Order an additional 100 cc sterile foley irrigation
c. Obtain a renal ultrasound
d. Obtain urine sodium and (fractional excretion of sodium) FE_{Na+} determination

4. A 45-year-old male presents to the outpatient clinic for a pre-employment physical examination. Laboratory findings are suggestive of renal insufficiency. The ACNP knows that renal insufficiency:

a. Represents 50% nephron loss
b. Is usually asymptomatic
c. Is reversible with early detection and treatment
d. Results in a compensatory increase in glomerular filtration rate (GFR)

5. Renal failure occurs when there is a decrease in renal function with a resultant retention of urea nitrogen and creatinine in the blood. A variety of physiologic insults can cause this decrease in function, and are classified as one of three types; prerenal, intrarenal, and postrenal. Differentiating the type is necessary to identify appropriate treatment. Which of the following is characteristic of postrenal failure?

a. It can be reversed when the underlying cause of hypoperfusion is corrected
b. It damages the epithelial basement membrane which can regenerate
c. It progresses to intrarenal failure in several days
d. It occurs due to mechanical or functional urine flow obstruction

6. Knowledge of sexually transmitted diseases (STD) is important for the ACNP regardless of practice site as STD represents a significant health condition for millions of Americans. The most common bacterial sexually transmitted disease in the U.S. is:

a. Gonorrhea
b. Herpes
c. Chlamydia
d. Syphilis

7. A 32-year-old male presents complaining of penile discharge. He is very concerned because last weekend he attended a bachelor party and was unfaithful to

his wife for the first and only time. The ACNP examines a smear of the discharge and finds gram negative diplococci and polymorphonuclear leukocytes. Given the history and clinical findings, the ACNP counsels the patient that he must tell his wife immediately because he likely has a condition that:

    a. Is the leading cause of infertility in U.S. females
    b. Will require 14 to 28 days of antibiotic treatment
    c. Frequently produces profound symptoms in women
    d. Requires treatment of all contacts

8. Which of the following statements is not true regarding herpes?

    a. It is a viral, sexually transmitted disease
    b. It is curable with early detection and prompt antibiotic treatment
    c. It is associated with painful genital lesions
    d. It is transmitted through direct contact with virus containing fluid or lesions

9. While working in the outpatient clinic, the ACNP encounters a 42-year-old female with a history of syphilis. She is complaining of a headache and stiff neck for the past three days. What stage of syphilis might be suspected?

    a. Primary
    b. Secondary
    c. Latent
    d. Tertiary

10. A 54-year-old male presents to an urgent care center where he is seen by an ACNP. He has no significant past medical history. He has been experiencing severe flank pain for two days, is currently afebrile, and denies urgency or hesitancy. A urinalysis reveals < 10 WBC/HPF.

The most likely diagnosis is:

    a. Cystitis
    b. Pyelonephritis
    c. Renal artery stenosis
    d. Renal calculi

11. You are the ACNP in the emergency department. A middle aged male presents with excruciating flank pain and nausea with vomiting. The KUB reveals a 4 mm diameter ureteral stone. Based on this finding the appropriate action would be:

a. Referral for lithotripsy
b. Intravenous pyelography (IVP) to assess for obstruction
c. Analgesia and hydration
d. Serum and urine blood tests to assess stone mineral type

12. A 46-year-old male presents with a sudden onset of renal insufficiency. Renal artery stenosis is suspected. Which of the following statements is not true regarding renal artery stenosis?

a. Renal artery stenosis is progressive and can lead to loss of renal function
b. Compensatory, contralateral hypertrophy may temporarily maintain renal function
c. Renal artery stenosis should be suspected when hypertension develops in a previously normotensive client
d. A negative captopril test is diagnostic of renal artery stenosis

13. Renal failure can result from prerenal, renal, and postrenal etiologies. Prerenal failure is most commonly caused by:

a. Nephrotoxicity
b. Acute tubular necrosis
c. Hypoperfusion
d. Urine flow obstruction

14. Mr. P. is a 63-year-old male who presents to the outpatient clinic with frequency, urgency, and leakage of urine for the past month. Which of the following should not be included in the differential diagnosis?

a. Prostate cancer
b. Benign prostatic hypertrophy
c. Acute bacterial prostatitis
d. Epididymitis

15. A 32-year-old female presents with suspected acute pyelonephritis. The most common causative organism of acute pyelonephritis is:

a. *Staphylococcus aureus*
b. *Escherichia coli*
c. *Enterococcus faecalis*
d. *Pseudomonas species*

Answers and Rationale

1. **(c)** Pyelonephritis is an upper urinary tract infection of the renal parenchyma. Characteristic findings include flank, low back or abdominal pain, fever, chills, and white blood casts seen on urinalysis (Carey, et al., p. 275).

2. **(c)** Patients with suspected pyelonephritis who can not tolerate oral antibiotic therapy, are pregnant, or have more severe illness (possible urosepsis) should be hospitalized for parenteral therapy until afebrile (24 to 72 hours). Outpatient treatment for patients who can tolerate oral antibiotics is a 14 day course (Carey, et al., p. 275).

3. **(d)** Urine sodium and fractional excretion of sodium (FE_{Na+}) determination can differentiate a prerenal from an intrarenal cause of oliguria. Prerenal failure is due to diminished blood flow and there is no nephron damage present. The conservation of sodium is maintained and urine sodium levels are low (< 20 mmol/dL) and the FE_{Na+} is low (< 1%). In intrarenal failure, nephron damage has occurred impairing the normal absorption and secretion ability of the tubules. Urine sodium levels are elevated (> 40 mmol/dL) and the FE_{Na+} is elevated (> 3%), indicating impairment in sodium reabsorption due to tubular damage (Marino, pp. 619-623).

4. **(b)** Patients are often asymptomatic until the late stages of renal insufficiency due to the compensatory ability of functioning nephrons. Renal insufficiency represents 75% nephron loss and is irreversible, but progression can be slowed with early diagnosis and treatment. Renal insufficiency results in a decreased glomerular filtration rate (Uphold & Graham, pp. 425-427).

5. **(d)** Postrenal failure occurs due to mechanical or functional urine flow obstruction. If untreated, postrenal failure can progress to intrarenal failure with the time frame being dependent on the degree, mechanism, and duration of obstruction (Carey, et al., p. 228-232).

6. **(c)** Chlamydia is the most common bacterial sexually transmitted disease in the United States (Uphold & Graham, pp. 649-651).

7. **(d)** Gonorrhea is a sexually transmitted bacterial infection which is a leading cause of infertility in U.S. females, but not the leading cause. Gonorrhea is

often asymptomatic but can produce dysuria and vaginal discharge. All contacts should be treated and cases reported to the health department. Uncomplicated gonorrhea is treated with any one of several single dose antibiotic regimens (Graber, et al., p. 499).

8. **(b)** Herpes is a viral, sexually transmitted disease with no cure. It is associated with painful genital lesions which are spread through direct contact with virus containing fluid or active lesions (Uphold & Graham, pp. 654-657).

9. **(d)** Tertiary syphilis should be suspected as the patient has meningeal symptoms (Carey, et al., p. 276).

10. **(d)** The most likely diagnosis is renal calculi. More common in men with an average age of onset > 30 years, renal calculi often present with flank pain that is usually seen with increasing intensity, radiating downward to the groin or over the abdomen (Mladenovic, pp. 234-238).

11. **(c)** Analgesia and hydration are important initial treatment measures for renal calculi. If the stone is < 6 mm in diameter, observation for passage for a four week period is advised. Referral to a urologist is indicated if the stone does not pass within a four week period. If the stone is obstructing urine outflow or is accompanied by infection, removal is indicated (Carey, et al., pp. 242-243).

12. **(d)** Renal artery stenosis can be diagnosed with a positive captopril test. A captopril test is positive when an exaggerated increase in plasma renin activity results from the administration of captopril (Fauci, et al., p. 1559).

13. **(c)** Prerenal failure is due to diminished blood flow. By definition, an episode of acute renal failure is prerenal only if it is reversed when the underlying cause of hypoperfusion is corrected. Common causes of prerenal failure include decreased cardiac output due to shock, congestive heart failure, dysrhythmias, vasodilation (sepsis), and decreased blood volume (hemorrhage, dehydration, diarrhea, burns). Nephrotoxicity and acute tubular necrosis can result in intrarenal failure and urine flow obstruction can result in postrenal failure (Marino, pp. 619-621).

14. **(d)** Prostate cancer, benign prostatic hypertrophy, and acute bacterial prostatitis all would be considered in the differential diagnosis of an elderly male with frequency, urgency, and leakage of urine. Severe scrotal pain, relieved by elevation, and fever would be characteristic of epididymitis (Uphold & Graham, pp. 421-422).

15. **(b)** *Escherichia coli* accounts for up to 80% of all upper UTI infections (Wallach, p. 391).

References

Carey, C., Lee, H., & Woeltje, K. (1998). *The Washington manual of medical therapeutics*. Philadelphia: Lippincott-Raven.

Fauci, A., Braunwald, E., Isselbacher, K., Wilson, J., Martin, J., Kasper, D., Hauser, S., & Longo, D. (Eds.), (1998). *Harrison's principles of internal medicine* (14th ed.). NY: McGraw-Hill.

Graber, M., Toth, P., & Herting, R. (1997). *The family practice handbook*. St. Louis: Mosby.

Marino, P. (1998). *The ICU book (2nd ed.)*. Baltimore: Williams & Wilkins.

Mladenovic, J. (1995). *Primary care secrets*. St. Louis: Mosby.

Uphold, C., & Graham, M. (1994). *Clinical guidelines in adult health*. Gainesville, Florida: Barmarrae Books.

Wallach, J. (1998). *Handbook of interpretation of diagnostic tests*. Philadelphia: Lippincott-Raven.

Musculoskeletal Disorders

Lynn A. Kelso

Select one best answer to the following questions.

Questions 1 and 2 refer to the following scenario.

A 26-year-old female is complaining of severe right ankle pain and swelling that began suddenly two hours ago. Vital signs are BP 108/76 mm Hg, heart rate 114 bpm, resp 18 bpm, and temp 38.6° C. Past medical history is significant for multiple ankle sprains. She has NKDA and her only medication is oral contraceptive pills.

1. Initial orders should include blood cultures and:

    a. Urine cultures
    b. Bilateral ankle radiographs
    c. Synovial fluid aspirate
    d. Gonococcal smears

2. The patient has received IV antibiotics for six days. She remains febrile with continued ankle pain and swelling. The last arthrocentesis was 24 hours ago. Your next action should be to:

    a. Increase the antibiotic dose
    b. Obtain an orthopedic consult
    c. Order q12h arthrocentesis
    d. Repeat all cultures

Questions 3 and 4 refer to the following scenario.

A 36-year-old female is complaining of pain and tingling that radiates up her left arm. She first experienced symptoms two weeks ago with tingling of her left wrist, but she became worried when she began experiencing pain in her neck and chest.

3. The ACNP should first order:

    a. ECG, cardiac enzymes
    b. Carpal compression test
    c. Upper extremity radiographs
    d. Left upper extremity (LUE) electromyography

4. To relieve her left arm pain the best intervention is:

    a. P.R.N. sublingual nitroglycerin
    b. Night splinting of wrist and forearm
    c. Cortisone injection in the affected wrist
    d. To consult orthopedic surgery

5. A 52-year-old male is complaining of severe lower back pain. The most important diagnostic tool for evaluating his complaint is a:

    a. Thorough history and physical
    b. Complete set of spinal radiographs
    c. CT of the abdomen
    d. MRI of the spine

6. A 73-year-old female with a history of osteoarthritis is complaining of fatigue, lightheadedness, and dyspnea on exertion. Along with serum electrolytes and an ECG, the evaluation should include a(n):

    a. Echocardiogram
    b. Sputum C&S
    c. Guaiac stool
    d. Chest radiograph

7. A 62-year-old female with a history of systemic lupus erythematosus (SLE) has recently been weaned from ventilatory support to a 40% aerosol face mask. She had developed ARDS which required neuromuscular blockade and sedation to improve ventilation. Current medications include cefotaxime, methylprednisolone, and famotidine. During her rehabilitation she is continually complaining of extremity weakness and inability to stand. She does not complain of pain. EMGs are normal. Your next course is to:

    a. Increase famotidine
    b. Taper methylprednisolone
    c. Increase methylprednisolone
    d. Discontinue famotidine

8. A 54-year-old male being treated for renal insufficiency is on furosemide 80

mg IV b.i.d. He was awakened during the night with severe pain in his right foot localized to the 1st and 2nd metatarsophalangeal joints. The therapy of choice would be:

    a. Indomethacin and MSO_4
    b. Indomethacin and colchicine
    c. Ice, elevation of his right foot, and MSO_4
    d. Methylprednisolone and MSO_4

9. A 63-year-old female was admitted to the hospital with severe back pain. Her past medical history is significant for chronic atrial fibrillation, hypertension, and a hysterectomy for cervical cancer at age 51. An abdominal source of back pain has been ruled out. You then order a:

    a. Myelogram
    b. Lumbar puncture
    c. Spinal radiograph
    d. MRI of the spine

10. A 49-year-old male is complaining of severe neck pain with frequent muscle spasms, which increase in intensity any time that he coughs. Physical examination reveals upper extremity DTR of +1 and decreased bilateral forearm sensation. The ACNP should order:

    a. Ice compresses b.i.d.
    b. Physical therapy
    c. Ibuprofen 800 mg q12h
    d. Cervical traction and bedrest

Answers and Rationale

1. **(c)** This patient presents a picture consistent with nongonococcal acute bacterial arthritis. The most appropriate actions are to obtain blood cultures to rule out bacteremia and to aspirate the joint. Synovial fluid should be sent for cell count and for glucose. White blood cell count is frequently high, with the greatest majority being neutrophils, and the glucose is usually low with infection (Hellmann, pp. 814-815).

2. **(b)** Joints that do not respond to appropriate therapy and repeated arthrocentesis within 5 to 7 days should be considered for surgical drainage (Lefkowith, p. 463).

3. **(a)** Although this patient has symptoms compatible with carpal tunnel syndrome, chest pain is not a usual finding. Whenever new chest pain is present, particularly new onset chest pain, a cardiac origin should be ruled out (Goldman, p. 61).

4. **(b)** The treatment for carpal tunnel syndrome is to relieve pressure on the median nerve. Splinting the hand and forearm at night may help to relieve symptoms (Hellmann, p. 788).

5. **(a)** The most common mistake made when evaluating patients with lower back pain is not obtaining an adequate history and physical examination. Lower back pain is a manifestation of many processes and a thorough history and physical examination can lead the evaluation in specific directions (Hellmann, p. 785).

6. **(c)** Osteoarthritis is frequently treated with nonsteroidal anti-inflammatory medications. These need to be used with caution in the elderly because gastrointestinal bleeding associated with the use of NSAID is increased in this population. The patient's symptoms may represent anemia, and GI bleeding should be ruled out (Lefkowith, p. 468).

7. **(b)** Glucocorticoids may be associated with myopathies. Weakness is frequently symmetrical and involves proximal limb girdle muscles. Improvement occurs slowly after removal of the offending agents and with aggressive exercise (Lefkowith, pp. 459-460).

8. **(d)** The patient is exhibiting symptoms of acute gout which can be exacerbated with hyperuricemia precipitated by diuretics. Although NSAID are frequently used to treat acute gout, they should be avoided or used with extreme caution in patients with renal insufficiency. The best treatment option would be steroids, which often provide dramatic symptomatic relief. Opioids may also be required to relieve pain (Hellmann, pp. 777-779).

9. **(c)** Postmenopausal osteoporosis frequently becomes clinically evident about 10 years after menopause. The greatest loss is with trabecular bone which frequently leads to vertebral crush fractures. This would be evident with spinal radiographs (Dagogo-Jack, p. 450).

10. **(d)** A herniation of the cervical disks into the spinal canal causes pain that radiates to the arms. There are frequently muscle spasms associated with the pain and it is aggravated by maneuvers that increase intra-abdominal pressure such as coughing or sneezing. Decreased deep tendon reflexes may be seen as well as weakness in the forearms. Conservative therapy, including cervical traction and bedrest, is usually successful. Athough ibuprofen may help to alleviate pain, the dose given is not appropriate and should be 200 to 400 mg every 4 to 6 hours (Hellmann, pp. 782-783).

References

Dagogo-Jack, S. (1998). Mineral and metabolic bone diseases. In C. F. Carey, H. H. Lee, & K. F. Woeltje (Eds.), *The Washington manual of medical therapeutics* (29th ed., pp. 441-455). Philadelphia: Lippincott-Raven.

Goldman, L. (1998). Chest discomfort and palpitation. In A. S. Fauci, E. Braunwald, K. J. Isselbacher, J. D. Wilson, J. B. Martin, D. L. Kasper, S. L. Hauser, & D. L. Longo (Eds.), *Harrison's principles of internal medicine* (14th ed., pp. 58-65). NY: McGraw-Hill.

Hellmann, D. B. (1998). Arthritis and musculoskeletal disorders. In L. M. Tierney, Jr., S. J. McPhee, & M. A. Papadakis (Eds.), *Current medical diagnosis and treatment* (37th ed., pp. 774-823). Stamford, CT: Appleton & Lange.

Lefkowith, J. B., & Kahl, L. E. (1998). Arthritis and rheumatologic diseases. In C. F. Carey, H. H. Lee, & K. F. Woeltje (Eds.), *The Washington manual of medical therapeutics* (29th ed., pp. 456-474). Philadelphia: Lippincott-Raven.

Common Problems in Acute Care

Candis Morrison

Select one best answer to the following questions.

Questions 1 and 2 refer to the following scenario.

Your patient is six hours post-laparoscopic cholecystectomy. Her temperature has risen from 36.4° C preoperatively to 39.5° C postoperatively.

1. The most likely cause of her fever is:

    a. Atelectasis
    b. Pneumonia
    c. IV site infection
    d. Wound infection

2. Initial measures in the treatment of this patient include:

    a. Antipyretics and oral hydration
    b. Hydration and measures to expand lung inflation
    c. Blood cultures and intravenous antibiotics
    d. Antipyretics and oral antibiotics

3. Which of the following conditions is not an indication to initiate empiric, broad spectrum antibiotic therapy in febrile patients?

    a. Temperature > 100.5° F
    b. Hemodynamic instability
    c. Neutropenia
    d. Concomitant use of systemic corticosteroids

4. When caring for an elderly patient with a fever it is important to consider that elderly patients may produce:

    a. A lesser response to pyrogenic stimuli than younger or middle aged adults

    b. A greater response to pyrogenic stimuli than younger or middle aged adults

    c. The same response to pyrogenic stimuli as younger or middle aged adults

    d. A delayed response to pyrogenic stimuli as compared to younger or middle aged adults

5. In most cases of hemorrhage leading to shock, the resultant acid-base imbalance would be:

    a. Respiratory acidosis

    b. Respiratory alkalosis

    c. Metabolic acidosis

    d. Metabolic alkalosis

6. When caring for a patient with acute respiratory acidosis, the ACNP remembers that an increase in $PaCO_2$ will:

    a. Decrease pH and decrease HCO_3^-

    b. Increase pH and increase HCO_3^-

    c. Increase pH and decrease HCO_3^-

    d. Decrease pH and increase HCO_3^-

7. When precise measurements of oxygenation are required, which two tests are necessary to evaluate acid-base status?

    a. Arterial blood gases and serum creatinine

    b. Arterial blood gases and serum electrolytes

    c. Serum electrolytes and pulse oximetry

    d. Pulse oximetry and serum lactate

8. A patient with ethylene glycol intoxication would most likely exhibit:

    a. Metabolic alkalosis with a normal anion gap

    b. Metabolic acidosis with an increased anion gap

    c. Respiratory alkalosis with a decreased anion gap

    d. Respiratory acidosis with a normal anion gap

9. Most pulmonary disorders cause respiratory acidosis. Which of the following conditions are associated with respiratory alkalosis secondary to hypoxemia?

    a. Atelectasis and pulmonary embolism

    b. Pneumothorax and airway obstruction

c. Depression of respiratory center secondary to narcotics
d. Chronic obstructive lung disease

10. Which of the following conditions would cause a normal anion gap acidosis?

a. Alcoholic ketoacidosis
b. Gastrointestinal HCO_3^- loss
c. Uremic acidosis
d. Lactic acidosis

11. A patient with chronic respiratory acidosis secondary to COPD is admitted with acute respiratory failure. Mechanical ventilation is intitiated. During the period in which his kidneys are compensating, you would expect to see:

a. Increased pH and increased bicarbonate
b. Increased pH and decreased bicarbonate
c. Decreased pH and increased bicarbonate
d. Decreased pH and decreased bicarbonate

12. A 19-year-old college student presents to the emergency department complaining of lightheadedness, anxiety, stocking and glove distribution paresthesias, and perioral numbness. She has a history of panic disorder. Chest radiograph is normal and her arterial blood gases reveal a low $PaCO_2$. The first intervention indicated to correct her acid base disorder is to:

a. Administer O_2 at 6 L/minute via nasal cannula
b. Administer sodium bicarbonate IV
c. Have her rebreathe into a paper bag
d. Have her take rapid shallow breaths

13. A patient with a long history of congestive heart failure has been on loop diuretics for six years. He recently experienced three days of nausea and vomiting that he attributed to food poisoning. Today he presents with weakness, hypotension, and decreased skin turgor. ABG reveals a pH of 7.47 and an elevated serum bicarbonate. Therapy should include infusion of:

a. HCO_3^-
b. D_5W
c. Colloids
d. Normal saline

14. In an apparent suicide attempt, a 22-year-old female ingested 16 acetamino-
    phen tablets four hours ago. Her serum acetaminophen level is 250 μg/mL.
    The appropriate antidote for this overdose is:

    a. Naloxone
    b. Flumazenil
    c. Sodium thiosulfate
    d. N-acetylcysteine

15. A 29-year-old secretary presents to the emergency department reporting that
    she ingested 40 aspirin tablets 20 minutes ago. She is alert and oriented and in
    no distress. The ACNP would order:

    a. Oral antacid, 30 cc p.o.
    b. Activated charcoal 50 g IV
    c. Sodium thiosulfate 250 mg/kg IV
    d. Syrup of ipecac 30 mL p.o.

16. An unidentified male is brought to the emergency department by friends. He is
    stuporous and confused. On examination he has pinpoint pupils and is hypoten-
    sive. He has track marks on both arms. Shortly after admission, he loses con-
    sciousness and experiences respiratory arrest. The ACNP would order:

    a. Diazepam
    b. Haloperidol
    c. Flumazenil
    d. Naloxone

17. A patient is brought to the emergency department status post overdose of an un-
    known substance. On initial examination her pupils are pinpoint. Her heart rate
    is 46 bpm and her BP is 90/40 mm Hg. She is drooling copiously and has been
    incontinent of urine and stool. What classification of ingested substance do you
    suspect?

    a. Opioid
    b. Amphetamine
    c. Benzodiazepine
    d. Cholinergic

18. A 59-year-old male is admitted to the emergency department after reportedly in-
    gesting 52 atenolol tablets 90 minutes ago. He is currently alert, but brady-
    cardic. What is the appropriate initial intervention?

    a. Induce emesis

   b. Ensure airway
   c. Administer antidote
   d. Administer activated charcoal

19. A 19-year-old college sophomore is admitted to the emergency department. History reveals that he consumed fifteen, 12 oz. beers over the course of two hours while participating in a party drinking game. Vital signs on admission include a temp of 37.2° C, heart rate of 112 bpm, resp of 10 bpm, and BP of 90 mm Hg palpable. He is difficult to arouse. He weighs approximately 70 kg. Which of the following treatment plans is most appropriate?

   a. Administer disulfiram intravenously
   b. Allow the patient to "sleep it off" in a holding room
   c. Insert a nasogastric (NG) tube and evacuate gastric contents
   d. Admit for CNS and respiratory monitoring

20. A 23-year-old presents with a four day old abscess in his left forearm. The arm is tender, warm, indurated, and erythematous. He has systemic symptoms of fever and fatigue. The mass is fluctuant and well encapsulated. The primary treatment would include:

   a. Incision and drainage
   b. Elevation and compression
   c. Ice and splinting
   d. Corticosteroids and antibiotics

Questions 21 and 22 refer to the following scenario.

A 34-year-old male is brought to the emergency department with a 4 cm clean, deep laceration on the dorsum of his foot, sustained by a lawn mower blade. His past health history is negative for chronic illness.

21. In preparation for suturing, it would be appropriate to:

   a. Soak the foot in 100% betadine solution and debride wound edges
   b. Shave the area around the laceration and soak in 10% betadine solution
   c. Vigorously scrub the wound before anesthesia is injected
   d. Clean the periphery with 1% betadine solution and then irrigate

22. Under which of the following conditions would this patient require immediate antibiotic therapy?

   a. It has been over three hours since the injury occurred

  b. His tetanus status is unknown
  c. He has a history of an infected wound five years ago
  d. You suspect a partially lacerated tendon

Questions 23 and 24 refer to the following scenario.

J. S. is a 50-year-old male brought to the emergency department after sustaining burns to his entire right arm, right leg, and the right side of the thorax and abdomen. These are all 2nd or 3rd degree burns.

23. What is the best estimate of percentage of his body that is burned?

  a. 27%
  b. 36%
  c. 45%
  d. 54%

24. As the ACNP you are concerned about tetanus prophylaxis in this patient. He recalls getting a tetanus shot when he cut his arm at work nine years ago. You would order:

  a. Tetanus toxoid 0.5 cc
  b. Td (tetanus and diptheria toxoids) 0.5 cc
  c. DPT (diptheria, pertussus and tetanus toxoids) 0.5 cc
  d. TIG (tetanus immune globulin) 250 U

Questions 25 and 26 refer to the following scenario:

A 43-year-old male is admitted to the medical intensive care unit (MICU). He has a history of nausea, vomiting, and anorexia. Past history is positive for hypertension controlled on beta blockers, and tobacco use. Vital signs are as follows: Temp 36.2° C, heart rate 80 bpm, resp 20 bpm, and BP 140/100 mm Hg. He is lethargic, confused and has bilateral, pitting tibial edema. Chest examination reveals bilateral crackles. Heart sounds are normal. He has 4 cm of JVD bilaterally. His DTRs are decreased throughout and he has a urine output of less than 10 mL per hour. Laboratory evaluation demonstrates a serum Na^+ of 132 mEq/L, a serum K^+ of 3.2 mEq/L, a serum osmolality of 245 mosm/L, and a urine Na^+ of > 20 mEq/L.

25. This clinical picture is most consistent with:

  a. Syndrome of inappropriate antidiuretic hormone
  b. Diabetes insipidus

c. Hypercalcemia
d. Addison's disease

26. Initial treatment for this condition may include:

a. Chlorpropamide
b. Thiazide diuretics
c. Fluid restriction
d. 500 cc bolus of normal saline solution

Questions 27 and 28 refer to the following scenario.

Your head injured patient has had 400 mL per hour urine output over the last four hours. The specific gravity is 1.002. A recent chemistry panel revealed a serum glucose of 96 mg/dL.

27. Which diagnosis is most consistent with this clinical scenario?

a. Diabetes mellitus
b. Diabetes insipidus
c. Syndrome of inappropriate antidiuretic hormone
d. Addison's disease

28. Intravenous (IV) fluid replacement most appropriate for this patient is:

a. Normal saline
b. Ringer's lactate
c. D_5W
d. 3% saline

29. A 43-year-old patient was admitted to the medical intensive care unit (MICU) with symptoms of intense thirst and polyuria, (reportedly ingesting > 10 L per day). He also complains of dizziness, muscle cramps, headaches, weight loss, and fatigue. On examination he has dry mucous membranes, poor skin turgor, and postural hypotension. Preadmission laboratory evaluation demonstrated a serum sodium of 152 mEq/L, with a serum osmolality of 300 mosm/L. Urine osmolality was < 10 mosm/L and urine specific gravity was also low. Urine glucose was negative. You would suspect:

a. Diabetes mellitus
b. Diabetes insipidus
c. Syndrome of inappropriate antidiuretic hormone
d. Cushing's syndrome

30. You are admitting a patient with acute adrenal insufficiency. Electrolyte abnormalities expected in this condition include:

    a. Hypokalemia, hyponatremia, and low blood urea nitrogen
    b. Hypokalemia, hypernatremia and low blood urea nitrogen
    c. Hyperkalemia, hyponatremia, and hyperglycemia
    d. Hyperkalemia, hyponatremia and hypoglycemia

Questions 31 and 32 refer to the following scenario.

A 63-year-old patient is admitted with a recent onset of nausea, vomiting, diarrhea, and new onset of confusion. Past medical history is positive for seizures. Physical findings include a heart rate of 110 bpm, supine BP of 110/80 mm Hg, upright BP of 90/58 mm Hg, and poor skin turgor. Serum electrolytes reveal a serum Na^+ of 128 mEq/L.

31. Which laboratory examination should be the next step in evaluating the cause of the sodium imbalance?

    a. Serum osmolality
    b. Serum osmolarity
    c. Urine catecholamines
    d. Urine sodium

32. An important complication of inadequately treated acute hyponatremia in this patient would be:

    a. Central diabetes insipidus
    b. Cerebral dehydration
    c. Cerebral embolus
    d. Cerebral edema

Questions 33 and 34 refer to the following scenario:

A 79-year-old male is brought to the ED complaining of shortness of breath of one day's duration and a two day history of nausea, vomiting, and weakness. He has been unable to pass urine for the past 18 hours. Past medical history is positive for atrial fibrillation, COPD, and benign prostatic hypertrophy (BPH). Medications include digoxin and coumadin. Vital signs include a temp of 38.2° C, heart rate of 126 bpm, resp of 28 bpm, BP of 118/60 mm Hg, and an O_2 saturation of 92%. 2L of O_2 are administered per nasal cannula and he is attached to the cardiac monitor.

It demonstrates sinus tachycardia with prolonged P-R intervals and wide QRS complexes which are irregularly placed. As suspected, his K^+ is elevated at 7.5 mEq/L.

33. Which underlying condition is the most likely cause of the hyperkalemia?

    a. Metabolic acidosis secondary to chronic hypoperfusion
    b. Respiratory acidosis secondary to COPD
    c. Reduced potassium excretion secondary to BPH
    d. Metabolic alkalosis secondary to vomiting

34. A foley catheter was placed and furosemide started. Because the hyperkalemia is severe, additional treatment may be indicated. Which of the following is not advantageous in this situation?

    a. Intravenous glucose
    b. Intravenous insulin
    c. Intravenous spironolactone
    d. Intravenous loop diuretics

35. A 65-year-old alcoholic male is found to have a serum Ca^{++} of 8.5 mEq/dL. He is carefully questioned regarding symptoms of the disorder and reports generalized muscle cramps and paresthesias around his lips. Which additional laboratory value would you need to rule out a calcium abnormality?

    a. Albumin
    b. Globulin
    c. Glucose
    d. Potassium

36. A 72-year-old woman presents complaining of nausea, polyuria, and constipation. Her muscles are weak upon examination and she exhibits depressed deep tendon reflexes. She has been supplementing her diet with calcium antacids in an effort to prevent osteoporosis. Her serum Ca^{++} is 11 mEq/dL. Serum albumin is normal. In an effort to correct the calcium you would begin treatment with:

    a. Hypotonic saline with thiazide diuretics
    b. Normal saline with loop diuretics
    c. Colloids and magnesium
    d. Normal saline and insulin

37. Patients on ACE inhibitors should be monitored for which two adverse effects of these drugs?

    a. Hyperkalemia and proteinuria
    b. Hypokalemia and thrombocytopenia
    c. Nephrotoxicity and congestive heart failure
    d. Atrial fibrillation and hyponatremia

Questions 38 and 39 refer to the following scenario.

A 63-year-old is brought to the urgent care center by her daughter. It is reported that over the course of the past two days she has become increasingly anxious. She is awake all night and seems drowsy during the day. On examination she is irritable, anxious, and pacing around the room. She denies a problem with her memory, though her daughter states that she is extremely forgetful. Her past medical history is negative, with the exception of a CVA three years ago. Physical examination is unremarkable. She scores 20 on a Folstein mini-mental status examination and is having extreme difficulty attending.

38. The ACNP strongly suspects this constellation of symptoms and signs to be due to:

    a. The normal effects of aging
    b. Malingering
    c. Hyperglycemia
    d. Delirium

39. Which medication is the safest choice for symptom relief?

    a. Amytriptyline
    b. Haloperidol
    c. Clonidine
    d. Lorazepam

40. An 84-year-old woman is hospitalized for a hip fracture. Her cognitive abilities have deteriorated over the course of her lengthy hospitalization. The differentiation between delirium and dementia is based on the:

    a. Age of the patient
    b. Response to neuroleptic medications
    c. Chronicity of the symptoms
    d. Severity of the symptoms

41. A 32-year-old male is admitted with the diagnosis of acute confusional state.

Symptom onset was sudden and associated with visual hallucinations and psychomotor restlessness. Physical examination reveals tachycardia, dilated pupils and diaphoresis. An important component of his initial evaluation is a:

a. Dexamethasone suppression test
b. Toxicology screen
c. 12 lead ECG
d. Gadolinium scan

Answers and Rationale

1. **(a)** Diffierential diagnosis of postoperative fever can be narrowed down by considering the time relationship of the onset of the fever to the surgery. Atelectasis is the most frequent cause of fever during the first 24 hours postoperatively secondary to decreased inflation of alveoli (Ganz, pp. 96-97).

2. **(b)** In the absence of any indication of infection, the first response to postoperative fever should include hydration and measures to expand lung inflation (Ganz, pp. 96-97).

3. **(a)** Most fever is well tolerated. Mild elevations only require fluid replacement. Empiric antibiotic therapy is only indicated in cases with high concurrent risk factors, such as comorbid immunosuppression (McPhee & Schroeder, pp. 25-27).

4. **(a)** Elderly patients tend to have lower baseline temperatures and often produce less impressive fever repsonse to pyrogenic stimuli than younger patients. Low grade fevers may be more significant (Daly & Glew, p. 177).

5. **(c)** Hemorrhagic shock causes increased peripheral lactic acid production. As liver perfusion declines, there is also a decreased hepatic metabolism of lactate. These factors contribute to the metabolic acidosis. In addition, severe acidosis impairs the ability of the liver to extract the perfused lactate. This is an increased anion gap acidosis (Okuda, et al., p. 842-843).

6. **(d)** Acute changes in $PaCO_2$ will cause a decrease in pH by 0.08 and an increase in HCO_3^- by 1 mEq/L (Ferri, p. 187).

7. **(b)** To adequately assess a patient's acid-base status, arterial pH, $PaCO_2$ and serum bicarbonate are required. The two tests to order are therefore ABG and serum electrolytes (Okuda, et al., p. 839).

8. **(b)** Multiple toxins and drugs can increase the anion gap by increasing endogenous acid production. Methanol (metabolized from formic acid), ethylene glycol (glycolic and oxalic acid), and salicylates (salicylic acid and lactic acid) are examples (Okuda, et al., pp. 842-844).

9. **(a)** Respiratory acidosis results from decreased alveolar ventilation and resulting hypercapnia. Respiratory alkalosis, or hypocapnia, occurs when hyperventilation decreases the $PaCO_2$, thus increasing the pH. The most common cause is hyperventilation syndrome. It can also be secondary to interstitial lung disease, pulmonary embolism, pulmonary edema, and atelectasis (Okuda, et al., pp. 839-841).

10. **(b)** The hallmark of normal anion gap acidosis is the low HCO_3^- of metabolic acidosis associated with hyperchloremia, so that the anion gap remains normal. The most common causes are gastrointestinal HCO_3^- loss with diarrhea. Bicarbonate is secreted in multiple areas in the GI tract. Diarrhea can result in HCO_3^- loss because of increased HCO_3^- secretion and decreased absorption (Ferri, p. 188).

11. **(a)** When chronic respiratory acidosis is corrected quickly, as with mechanical ventilation, there is a 2 to 3 day lag in renal bicarbonate excretion resulting in posthypercapnic metabolic alkalosis (Okuda, et al., p. 848).

12. **(c)** Hyperventilation is the likely etiology for these symptoms, particularly in an individual with an anxiety/panic disorder. Treatment is directed toward the underlying cause. In acute hyperventilation syndrome from anxiety, rebreathing into a paper bag will increase $PaCO_2$. If unsuccessful, sedation may be required (Okuda, et al., p. 841).

13. **(d)** This clinical picture is consistent with metabolic alkalosis from volume contraction. Diuretics and decreased fluid intake are common precipitators. This disorder should respond to saline and the therapy includes correction of the extracellular volume deficit. Adequate amounts of 0.9% NaCl and KCl should be administered, and diuretics discontinued pending normalization (Okuda, et al., pp. 847-848).

14. **(d)** The specific antidote for acetaminophen is N-acetylcysteine. It is dosed at 140 mg/kg and is most effective when administered in the first 16 hours after ingestion. The antidote is recommended if the serum level exceeds the toxic line on the nomogram for prediction of hepatotoxicity following acute overdose (Olson, pp. 1474-1475).

15. **(d)** Gastric emptying of substances ingested less than one hour prior to treatment is probably beneficial unless the patient is obtunded or comatose, has ingested a caustic substance, or ingested phenothiazines or petroleum products (Weinstock, p. 106).

16. **(d)** This case is suggestive of narcotic overdose, probably heroin. Treatment is naloxone, 2 mg IV. Results are evident within two minutes and are quite dramatic (Eisendrath, p. 1019).

17. **(d)** This patient is exhibiting parasympathetic signs such as those seen secondary to organophosphate poisoning. These act as anticholinesterase agents. Patients present in coma with pinpoint pupils. They may exhibit fasiculations. The antidote for this poisoning is atropine 0.5 to 2 mg IV. Atropine physiologically blocks acetylcholine (Weinstock, p. 113).

18. **(b)** The initial consideration in any overdose is emergency stabilization. It is crucial to ensure adequate ventilation and examine the airway for patency and intact gag reflex. Clearing the toxin is secondary (Weinstock, p. 103).

19. **(d)** This patient reveals signs of acute intoxication. A 12 oz. bottle of beer raises the blood alcohol level by 25 mg/dL in a 70 kg person. Lethal blood levels are in the range from 350 to 900 mg/dL. This patient requires close monitoring for acute alcohol overdosage leading to respiratory depression, seizures, and/or shock (Eisendrath, p. 1016).

20. **(a)** The lesion described in the scenario is one that requires surgical drainage. Antibiotics are frequently prescribed concurrently (Bartlett, pp. 622-623).

21. **(d)** Research has demonstrated that soaking cannot penetrate beyond 1.5 mm tissue and significant contamination may result. Shaving can increase the wound infection rate. There is no evidence that needles can spread bacteria beyond wound margins, so most wounds should be anesthetized before cleaning. 1% betadine solution can be safely applied to wounds and retains its bactericidal activity at this concentration. Dirty wounds should be irrigated (Trott, pp. 90-92).

22. **(d)** Suspected penetration of bone, joints, or tendons is an indication for immediate antibiotic therapy, particularly in a distal extremity (Trott, p. 129).

23. **(c)** The "rule of nines" is commonly used for estimating burn size in adults. Each arm is 9%, each leg 18%. The entire thorax and abdomen (anterior and posterior) is 36%. Since one half was affected, you add 18% + 9% + 18% = 45%. First degree burns are not included in these calculations (Trott, p. 305).

24. **(b)** The currently recommended CDC regimen is tetanus toxoid combined with the diptheria toxoid. The risk of contracting diptheria in adulthood is still of significant magnitude to justify prophylaxis (Trott, pp. 359-360).

25. **(a)** The diagnosis of SIADH is made only if the patient is euvolemic since increased ADH secretion is physiologic in hypovolemic states. SIADH is characterized by hyponatremia, decreased osmolality (< 280 mosm/kg) with inappropriately increased urine osmolality (> 150 mosm/kg), urine sodium usually over 20 mEq/L and absence of cardiac, renal, liver, and thyroid disorders (Okuda, et al., pp. 826-827).

26. **(c)** Initial treatment of SIADH is restriction of total water intake, usually to one liter or less per day. With this regimen, the hyponatremia and all other features of the disorder will resolve. The medications that are mentioned can acutally induce SIADH (Lafayette, pp. 243-294).

27. **(b)** Classic signs and symptoms of DI include diuresis of very dilute urine with normal serum glucose. The history of head injury is a clue to the diagnosis (Lafayette, pp. 249-250).

28. **(c)** Since hypernatremia is common with DI, you should infuse D_5W. The other three solutions would contribute to hypernatremia (Lafayette, p. 550).

29. **(b)** The diagnosis of DI as a cause of polyuria requires mostly clinical judgment. DM is ruled out by the negative urine glucose. Cushing's syndrome also causes hyperglycemia which results from the inability of glucose to be taken up by the cells. SIADH would cause hyponatremia (Fitzgerald, pp. 1037-1038).

30. **(d)** Acute adrenal insufficiency is an emergent condition caused by insufficient adrenal hormones. Cortisol counters the effects of insulin and tends to

cause hyperglycemia. Lack of cortisol would thus cause hypoglycemia. Aldosterone stimulates the renal tubule to reabsorb sodium and excrete potassium, thereby protecting against hypovolemia and hyperkalemia which are the electrolyte abnormalities seen when there is an aldosterone deficiency (Fitzgerald, pp. 1072-1073).

31. **(d)** The most direct and practical approach to the patient with hyponatremia is to evaluate the urine sodium. It is only necessary to measure serum osmolality when pseudohyponatremia or hyperosmolar conditions are suspected. A urine sodium of < 20 mEq/L suggests that the hyponatremia is secondary to the vomiting and diarrhea. If it were > 20 mEq/L, other causes would require investigation, such as osmotic diuresis, salt losing nephropathy, adrenal insufficiency, and excessive use of diuretics (Lafayette, pp. 239-241).

32. **(d)** Patients with symptomatic, severe, acutely developed hyponatremia require emergency treatment. Low osmolality of extracelluar fluid causes movement of water into relatively hypertonic brain neurons and can cause cerebral edema. This may progress to obtundation, coma and cerebral herniation (Burrow & Kauffman, p. 369).

33. **(c)** Renal potassium excretion will increase in response to serum hyperkalemia, therefore transcellular shifts are generally mild. Serum potassium concentration rarely exceeds 6.0 mEq/L unless there is a simultaneous reduction in renal potassium excretion. This patient's history of BPH and his inability to void have produced this picture. Mild respiratory acidosis would cause no significant rise in serum potassium concentration, nor would acute lactic acidosis (Lafayette, p. 261).

34. **(c)** Severe hyperkalemia ($K^+ > 6$ mEq/L) with ECG abnormalities is treated more aggressively. If the ECG shows QRS widening, it is essential to administer 10 mL of 10% calcium gluconate IV, immediately, to prevent malignant dysrhythmias; the calcium dose may be repeated every 15 minutes. This reverses the effect of the hyperkalemia on cell membranes. Dextrose and insulin may be administered to shift the potassium into the intracellular fluid and loop diuretics are used to remove potassium from the body. Dialysis is used if the above therapies are not corrective. Potassium sparing diuretics are definitely containdicated (Lafayette, pp. 265-266).

35. **(a)** The depressed level of serum calcium must be correlated with the simultaneous concentration of serum albumin. Albumin is the principle calcium-binding protein. Low albumin is correlated with depressed calcium in a ratio of 0.8 to 1 mg of calcium to one gram of albumin. The history of alcoholism could predispose to a hypoalbuminemic state (Okuda, et al., p. 833).

36. **(b)** This clinical picture is consistent with the milk-alkali syndrome associated with ingestion of calcium supplements used for osteoporosis. In this syndrome, massive calcium and Vitamin D ingestion can cause hypercalcemic nephropathy. Excretion of sodium is accompanied by excretion of calcium. Inducing calcium excretion by giving saline with furosemide is the emergency treatment of choice for hypercalcemia. Thiazides can worsen hypercalcemia as can loop diuretics if inadequate saline is given (Okuda, et al., p. 834).

37. **(a)** ACE inhibitors may cause hyperkalemia through inhibiting the secretion of aldosterone triggered by angiotensin II. Proteinuria may occur and even lead to nephrotic syndrome and renal failure. The practitioner needs to monitor serum K^+ and urine protein for these potential effects (Kimmelsteil & Konstam, pp. 69-70).

38. **(d)** Delirium or acute confusional state is a transient global disorder of attention, with clouding of consciousness. It is usually the result of systemic problems, such as drugs or hypoxia (Bell, pp. 692-693).

39. **(b)** Intravenous haloperidol has been proven to be the safest neuroleptic to use for the treatment of delirium. The incidence of dyskinesias has been low even at high dosage levels (McHugh, p. 921).

40. **(c)** Delirium is a transient global disorder of attention which is usually secondary to systemic problems. Dementia is characterized by chronicity and deterioration of selective mental functions (Eisendrath, p. 1024).

41. **(b)** Substance or alcohol withdrawl is the most common cause of delirium in the general hospital setting and is a treatable cause of delirium. A toxicology screen is required to confirm the diagnosis and specifically identify the substance (Eisendrath, p. 1024).

References

Bartlett, J. G. (1996). Infections of the skin, soft tissue and bone. In J. D. Stobo, D. B. Hellmann, P. W. Ladenson, B. G. Petty, & T. A. Traill (Eds.), *The principles and practice of medicine* (23rd ed.). Stamford, CT: Appleton & Lange.

Bell, I. R. (1996). Psychiatric conditions in the elderly. In H. L. Greene (Ed.), *Clinical medicine* (2nd ed.). St. Louis: Mosby.

Burrow, C. R., & Kauffman, M. G. (1996). Disorders of water and electrolyte balance. In J. D. Stobo, D. B. Hellmann, P. W. Ladenson, B. G. Petty, & T. A. Traill (Eds.), *The principles and practice of medicine* (23rd ed.). Stamford, CT: Appleton & Lange.

Daly, J. S., & Glew, R. H. (1996). Constitutional symptoms. In H. L. Greene (Ed.), *Clinical medicine* (2nd ed.). St. Louis: Mosby.

Eisendrath, S. J. (1998). Psychiatric disorders. In L. M. Tierney, Jr., S. J. McPhee, & M. A. Papadakis (Eds.), *Current medical diagnosis and treatment* (37th ed.). Stamford, CT: Appleton & Lange.

Ferri, F. (1998). Cardiovascular diseases. *Practical guide to the care of the medical patient* (4th ed.). St. Louis: Mosby.

Fitzgerald, P. A. (1998). Endocrinology. In L. M. Tierney, Jr., S. J. McPhee, & M. A. Papadakis (Eds.), *Current medical diagnosis and treatment* (37th ed.). Stamford CT: Appleton & Lange.

Ganz, N. M. (1997). Infectious disease. In J. T. Harrington (Ed.), *Consultant in internal medicine* (2nd ed.). St. Louis: Mosby.

Kimmelstiel, C. D., & Konstam, M. A. (1997). Management of congestive heart failure. In J. Harrington (Ed.), *Consultation in internal medicine* (2nd ed.). St. Louis: Mosby.

Lafayette, R. A. (1997). Hyponatremia and hyernatremia. In J. T. Harrington (Ed.). *Consultant in internal medicine* (2nd ed.). St. Louis: Mosby.

McHugh, P. R. (1996). Approach to the patient with a suspected psychiatric disorder. In J. D. Stobo, D. B. Hellmann, P. W. Ladenson, B. G. Petty, & T. A. Traill (Eds.), *The principles and practice of medicine* (23rd ed.). Stamford, CT: Appleton & Lange.

McPhee, S. J., & Schroeder, S. A. (1998). General approach to the patient: Health maintenance and disease prevention and common symptoms. In L. M. Tierney, Jr., S. J. McPhee, & M. A. Papadakis (Eds.), *Current medical diagnosis and treatment* (37th ed.). Stamford CT: Appleton & Lange.

Okuda, T., Kurokawa, K., & Papadakis, M.A. (1998). Fluid and electrolyte disorders. In L. M. Tierney, Jr., S. J. McPhee, & M. A. Papadakis (Eds.), *Current medical diagnosis and treatment* (37th ed.). Stamford, CT: Appleton & Lange.

Olson, K. R. (1998). Poisoning. In L. M. Tierney, Jr., S. J. McPhee, & M. A. Papadakis (Eds.), *Current medical diagnosis and treatment* (37th ed.). Stamford, CT: Appleton & Lange.

Trott, A. T. (1997). *Wounds and lacerations: Emergency care and closure* (2nd ed.). St Louis: Mosby.

Weinstock, M. S. (1998). General management of poisoning and drug overdose. In F. F. Ferri (Ed.), *Practical guide to the care of the medical patient* (4th ed.). St. Louis: Mosby.

Shock States/Trauma

Candis Morrison

Select one best answer to the following questions.

1. A 29-year-old male is brought to the trauma center by helicopter status post gun shot wound to the abdomen. Paramedics estimate that he has lost two liters of blood. His pulse is weak at 140 bpm and his blood pressure is palpable at 50 mm Hg. Skin is cool and extremities are cyanotic. Neck veins are completely flat. His chest is clear, and his heart sounds are weak. To prevent irreversible shock related complications while preparing him for the operating room, it is important to immediately infuse:

   a. Isotonic crystalloids through a short, large bore IV
   b. Colloids at a rate of 3 to 4 times the volume deficit
   c. Sodium bicarbonate to prevent metabolic acidosis
   d. Broad spectrum antibiotics to prevent sepsis

2. A 32-year-old woman is one day postoperative cardiac transplant for cardiomyopathy. Her mediastinal tube has been draining normally. Vital signs at 8 a.m. reveal a temp of 37.2° C, heart rate of 124 bpm, resp of 28 bpm, and BP of 90/50 mm Hg. Her skin is cold and clammy. There is 9 cm of JVD at 45 degrees and crackles in both bases. The best treatment for this patient is to:

   a. Treat infection with broad spectrum antibiotics
   b. Increase preload with fluid bolus
   c. Increase contractility with inotropic agents
   d. Decrease afterload with calcium channel blockers

3. The condition of a patient in the surgical ICU has just deteriorated. His blood pressure has dropped to 60/30 mm Hg and his heart rate has increased to 145 bpm. You observe that his jugular veins are visibly distended. Which type of shock is most consistent with these signs and symptoms?

   a. Hypovolemic
   b. Cardiogenic

    c. Septic

    d. Anaphylactic

4. You are called to the emergency department to admit a patient who is reportedly in shock. This blood pressure is palpable at 70 mm Hg and his heart rate is 160 bpm. On examination his extremities are pink and warm. This is consistent with which of the following shock states?

    a. Hypovolemic

    b. Cardiogenic

    c. Obstructive

    d. Distributive

5. A. P. is a 52-year-old patient with a history of HIV and Hodgkin's disease. She has completed her first cycle of chemotherapy and presents for admission for her second cycle. She is complaining of lethargy, weakness, anorexia, and fever. Her total white blood cell count is 500/μL with an absolute neutrophil count of 230/μL, and hemoglobin is 8 g/dL. Her temp is 39.8° C, heart rate 136 bpm, resp 32 bpm, and BP is palpable at 60 mm Hg. She is admitted and a pulmonary artery catheter is placed. Her cardiac output is 11 mL/min and the pulmonary artery wedge pressure is 5 mm Hg. Arterial blood gases reveal the following: pH 7.26, $PaCO_2$ 25 mm Hg, HCO_3^- 16 mEq/L, and PaO_2 64 mm Hg. This clinical picture is most consistent with which form of shock?

    a. Hypovolemic

    b. Anaphylactic

    c. Septic

    d. Neurogenic

6. A 19-year-old lifeguard is brought to the emergency department reporting that he was stung by a wasp at work 10 minutes ago. Because of his allergy history, he was brought to the emergency room immediately. While being registered he begins to wheeze and loses consciousness. BP is palpable at 110 mm Hg. The first action to take in this scenario is to:

    a. Start an IV and administer aminophylline

    b. Intubate and bag breathe until mechanical ventilation is initiated

    c. Administer 100 mg of hydrocortisone intravenously

    d. Inject epinephrine subcutaneously

7. Which of the following is a reliable diagnostic and prognostic indicator of shock states?

   a. Hemoglobin < 8 g/dL
   b. SaO$_2$ < 90%
   c. Serum lactate > 2.5 mmol/L
   d. Serum bicarbonate > 28 mEq/dL

8. E. G. is brought to the neurological critical care unit following emergency care for a head injury sustained in a fall from an eight foot ladder. His head reportedly hit a window sill and he immediately lost consciousness. Head CT has ruled out acute intracranial bleeding. He is hypotensive, tachycardic, and his skin is cool and clammy. He has no repsonse to pain. His Glascow coma score is 3. This patient is experiencing which type of shock?

   a. Hypovolemic
   b. Septic
   c. Cardiogenic
   d. Neurogenic

9. A patient is brought to the emergency department after a motor vehicle accident. He is diagnosed with respiratory distress. On examination his breath sounds are decreased on the right, and there is hyperresonance to percussion over the left lower lobe. Shortly after arrival his left breath sounds disappear and he begins to evidence signs of shock—tachycardia, hypotension and confusion. As the ACNP you immediately:

   a. Order a chest radiograph to determine need for a chest tube
   b. Order a chest CT to assess for pneumothorax
   c. Insert a needle in the second right intercostal space anteriorly
   d. Intubate immediately to prevent hypoxia

10. When evaluating a case of blunt abdominal trauma, indications for the need to perform peritoneal lavage include:

   a. Hypotension and pain
   b. Abdominal pain but stable vital signs
   c. An allergy to CT contrast dye
   d. Evidence of free air in the abdomen

11. A 39-year-old is brought to the emergency department after a three car collision in which he was a passenger. He is now alert and oriented, however he was unconscious when paramedics reached the accident scene. He is wearing a cervical collar and is asking you to remove it. The collar may be safely removed after:

    a. You complete a neurologic examination of the extremities
    b. C-1 to C-7 are radiographically visualized and declared normal
    c. Glascow coma score is ≥ 11
    d. Cranial CT reveals no evidence of cranial bleed

12. Rapidly reversible causes of CNS depression should be considered in all patients presenting with unexplained unconsciousness. They should receive:

    a. $D_{50}W$, thiamine, and naloxone
    b. Fluid bolus, epinephrine, and oxygen
    c. Oxygen, inotropes, and fluids
    d. Antibiotics, colloids, and oxygen

Answers and Rationale

1. **(a)** This patient is in hypovolemic shock due to rapid loss of blood. The mainstay of management of hypovolemic shock is rapid restoration of vascular volume. Animal models have demonstrated that, during the early phase of hypovolemic shock, cardiac output and arterial pressure can be returned to normal by administration of fluids in the first 90 minutes even when more than 40% of blood volume was rapidly lost. When isotonic saline is used, it is necessary to infuse 3 to 4 times the estimated lost volume. Smaller quantities of colloids are required to restore circulating blood volume (Brower & Fessler, p. 969).

2. **(c)** This patient exhibits clinical indications of pump failure and cardiogenic shock secondary to decreased contractility. This is best treated with inotropic agents (Roberts, p. 73).

3. **(b)** Unlike most forms of shock, cardiogenic shock is associated with increased jugular venous pressure and increased right atrial pressure. The decreased central venous pressure is seen with hypovolemic and distributive forms of shock (Brower & Fessler, pp. 968-72).

4. **(d)** In hypovolemic and cardiogenic shock, the circulating concentrations of catecholamines and angiotensins rise, producing vasoconstriction or cold shock. Distributive shock is manifested in an opposite manner as a consequence of the release of endotoxin and endogenous vasodilators. These produce peripheral vasodilation, or warm shock, in which the patient has warm extremities despite hypotension. Distributive shock is also known as high output shock (Effron & Chernow, p. 5).

5. **(c)** This patient's history and hemogram demonstrate risk for septic shock. Microbial pathogens trigger events involving exogenous and endogenous mediators that cause diffuse vascular inflammation, intravascular coagulation, and decreased vascular smooth muscle tone leading to loss of regulation of cardiac output and its distribution (Brower & Fessler, p. 971).

6. **(d)** Patients who present with anaphylaxis require immediate, subcutaneous aqueous 1:1000 epinephrine in a dose of 0.01 mg/kg. Intravenous access should then be established (Valentine, pp. 303-304).

7. **(c)** Blood lactate determinations have proved to be useful markers in shock patients. Studies have revealed that increased blood lactate values > 2.5 mmol/L are correlated with decreased oxygen delivery. Mortality is increased in patients with an increased serum lactate concentration (Effron & Chernow, p. 5).

8. **(a)** Isolated head injuries do not cause shock. The presence of shock in a patient with a head injury necessitates a search for another cause of shock. In this patient, the most likely cause would be hypovolemic shock secondary to intra-abdominal bleeding caused by the fall (Society of Critical Care Medicine, 1996b, pp. 69-73).

9. **(c)** This patient evidences signs of obstructive shock due to tension pneumothorax. This develops when a puncture in the visceral pleura functions as a valve, allowing air to be drawn into the pleural space during inspiration and preventing it from escaping during expiration. The resulting rise in pleural pressure compresses the heart and great veins, thus obstructing cardiac output. Management must be directed at restoration of the pressure gradient for venous return. Air in the chest should be evacuated quickly either through a chest tube or by inserting a large bore needle between two ribs (Brower & Fesslser, p. 972).

10. **(a)** Diagnostic peritoneal lavage is indicated in a patient with unexplained or refractory hypotension after blunt abdominal injury (Marx, p. 734).

11. **(b)** Injury to the cervical spine must be assumed to be present whenever consciousness is disturbed secondary to trauma. Five to ten percent of such patients will have a major cervical injury. Absolute immobilization of the C-spine is critical in patients presenting after trauma with even minor abnormalities of mental status, significant head or facial injuries, or other symptoms suggestive of cervical injury. Immobilization should be maintained until radiologic visualization of C-1 to C-7 is complete and determined to be normal (Society of Critical Care Medicine, 1996a, pp. 105-106).

12. **(a)** Hypoglycemia, opiate overdose, and Wernicke's encephalopathy must be considered initially and prophylactically treated in all patients with altered consciousness of unknown etiology. These are commonly precipitants of trauma (Fisher, pp. 827-828).

References

Alexander, R. H., & Proctor, H. J. (1993). Shock. *Advanced trauma life support course for physicians.* Chicago: American College of Surgeons.

Brower, R., & Fessler, H. E. (1996). Shock and multiple organ dysfunction syndrome. In J. D. Stobo, D. B. Hellmann, P. W. Ladenson, B. G. Petty, & T. A. Traill (Eds.), *The principles and practice of medicine* (23rd ed.). Stamford, CT: Appleton & Lange.

Effron, M. B., & Chernow, B. (1996) Shock. *Scientific American, 1*(3), 5.

Fisher, R. S. (1996). The unconscious patient. In J. D. Stobo, D. B. Hellmann, P. W. Ladenson, B. G. Petty, & T. A. Traill (Eds.), *The principles and practice of medicine* (23rd ed.). Stamford, CT: Appleton & Lange.

Marx, J. A. (1998). Peritoneal procedures. In J. R. Roberts, & J. R. Hedges (Eds.), *Clinical procedures in emergency medicine* (3rd ed.). Philadelphia: W. B. Saunders.

Roberts, S. (1996). Cardiac deviations. *Critical care nursing: Assessment and intervention.* Stamford, CT: Appleton & Lange.

Society of Critical Care Medicine. (1996a). Basic trauma management. *Fundamental critical care support.* Anaheim, CA: Society of Critical Care Medicine.

Society of Critical Care Medicine. (1996b). Diagnosis and management of shock. *Fundamental critical care support.* Anaheim, CA: Society of Critical Care Medicine.

Valentine, M. D. (1999). Allergy and related conditions. In L. R. Barker, J. R. Burton, & P. D. Zieve (Eds.), *Principles of ambulatory medicine* (5th ed.). Baltimore: Williams & Wilkins.

Pain and Immobility

Lynn A. Kelso

Select one best answer to the following questions.

Questions 1 and 2 refer to the following scenario.

A 57-year-old male is being treated for severe ARDS following an abdominal arotic aneurysm (AAA) repair. He is currently on a vecuronium drip at 4 mg/hr, MSO_4 drip at 2 mg/hr, and receiving lorazepam 4 mg IV q4h. His vital signs are BP 108/58 mm Hg, heart rate 128 bpm, resp 14/14 bpm, temp 36.8° C, CVP 12 mm Hg, PAP 30/18 mm Hg, PCWP 16 mm Hg, and SaO_2 96%.

1. Concerned about his tachycardia you:

    a. Start a continuous lorazepam drip
    b. Give 500 cc normal saline bolus
    c. Increase the MSO_4 drip
    d. Decrease the vecuronium drip

2. After weaning the above patient from his vecuronium, MSO_4, and lorazepam, you attempt to assess his neurological function. He remains sedated and is only responsive to noxious stimuli. The appropriate action would be to:

    a. Order a head CT scan
    b. Give 0.2 mg flumazenil IV
    c. Order an EEG
    d. Wait and reassess in 24 hours

3. A 21-year-old male status post cholecystectomy is complaining of incisional pain. He has received intermittent IM MSO_4 with minimal pain relief. To manage his pain the ACNP would order:

    a. Patient controlled analgesia (PCA) with MSO_4
    b. Oxycodone with acetaminophen p.o.
    c. Hydromorphone hydrochloride IV
    d. Acetaminophen p.o.

4. You are emergently paged to see a 63-year-old female who is on the floor 48 hours after a CABG. The staff informs you that she has become increasingly lethargic over the past eight hours and was found in bed responsive only to noxious stimulation. Vital signs are BP 94/60 mm Hg, heart rate 64 bpm, and resp 4 bpm. She is being adequately ventilated with 100% bag valve mask (BVM) and pulse oximeter readings are 98%. The first step should be:

   a. Emergent intubation
   b. Flumazenil 0.4 mg IV
   c. Naloxone 0.4 mg IV
   d. Atropine 1 mg IV

5. A 43-year-old male being treated for a metastatic brain tumor is continuing to complain of pain although he is receiving MSO_4 8 mg IV q2h. You respond by ordering:

   a. Lorazepam 4 mg IV q4h
   b. MSO_4 8 mg IV q1h
   c. Hydromorphone HCl 2 mg IV q1h
   d. Prednisone 20 mg p.o. b.i.d.

6. You are evaluating a 39-year-old patient with diabetes who is complaining of bilateral foot pain. There are no lesions or wounds on either foot and pulses are present with doppler. He is experiencing minimal relief from oxycodone HCl. You would then order:

   a. Phenytoin
   b. Codeine
   c. Prednisone
   d. Ibuprofen

7. A 54-year-old patient recovering from a total colectomy due to carcinoma is having increased pain. She is receiving MSO_4 4 mg IV p.r.n. The ACNP would order:

   a. Ibuprofen p.o.
   b. Ketorolac IV
   c. Acetaminophen p.r.
   d. Meperidine 50 mg IM

8. A 78-year-old male being treated for prostate cancer is on the following medications: Digoxin 0.25 mg p.o. q.d.; nifedipine SR 90 mg q.d.; oxycodone HCl

2 p.o. q4h. Although he states he has no other pain, he is complaining of abdominal cramping and has not had a bowel movement in three days. The ACNP should order:

   a. Fleets enema and MSO_4 4 mg IV
   b. Lactulose syrup
   c. Bisacodyl p.o. and reduction of oxycodone HCl
   d. Polyethylene glycol-electrolyte solution p.o. and fleets enema

9. A 73-year-old female has been on bedrest for three weeks at home. When attempting to get out of bed she became lightheaded and had to be helped back to bed by her caregiver. To prevent this the caregiver should:

   a. Increase the patient's fluid intake
   b. Position the patient as close to upright as possible t.i.d.
   c. Do passive range of motion exercises t.i.d.
   d. Sit the patient for five minutes prior to standing

10. The primary care nurse calls to tell you that a 53-year-old patient, who is on bedrest with cervical traction, has edema and tenderness of his left foot. You order:

   a. Bilateral duplex ultrasonography
   b. Arteriogram of lower extremities
   c. Heparin 5000 unit IV bolus
   d. Furosemide 40 mg IV

11. In a patient on bedrest, which of the following will increase the risk for developing a deep vein thrombosus (DVT)?

   a. Increased body surface area (BSA)
   b. Hypertension
   c. Coagulopathy
   d. Recent weight loss

12. An 82-year-old male has been on self-prescribed bedrest since the death of his wife. His son is concerned and has brought him into the hospital. The patient's past medical history is unremarkable and he is currently on no medications. He denies any pain. You consider ordering a:

   a. Head CT
   b. Psychology consult
   c. Neurology consult
   d. MRI of the spine

Answers and Rationale

1. **(c)** Because a patient who is paralyzed and sedated can not complain of increased pain, other signs must be assessed. This patient is tachycardic but the remainder of his vital signs are stable. He has adequate filling pressures so his tachycardia should be interpreted as an indication of pain. When other physiologic causes of tachycardia have been ruled out, pain must be considered in the patient with neuromuscular blockade. His drip should be increased and he should then be reassessed (Marino, p. 803).

2. **(b)** The patient was on a continuous infusion of opioids and benzodiazepines and there may be residual effects from the medications. Prior to ordering other diagnostic tests, mental status can be quickly assessed by reversing those agents. Flumazenil is a benzodiazepine antagonist (Goodenberger, p. 521).

3. **(a)** More reliable plasma opioid levels can be achieved with a PCA pump. Using a PCA also gives the patient more control over his pain. There is also increased patient satisfaction with PCA, and PCA is a popular form of pain control in awake, postoperative patients. Oral pain medications may be inadequate and cause nausea if the patient is NPO. Intermittent hydromorphone HCl may have no benefit over intermittent MSO_4 (McPhee, p. 23).

4. **(c)** Postoperative patients will have pain medication ordered. Dose dependent respiratory depression does occur with opioids, especially in patients with cardiac disease, thoracic and upper abdominal surgery, and in patients over the age of 70. Because the patient is being adequately ventilated with a BVM, an attempt can be made to reverse the opioids. If this is unsuccessful, the patient should be intubated and other causes of decreased level of consciousness should be assessed (McPhee, p. 23).

5. **(d)** Corticosteroids may be useful in managing cancer pain. They help to reduce cerebral edema and have a potent anti-inflammatory effect (McPhee, pp. 24-25).

6. **(a)** Anticonvulsant agents may help to control neuropathic pain (McPhee, p. 25).

7. **(b)** Nonsteroidal anti-inflammatory agents may be useful, in combination with opioids, to decrease pain. Because of the surgical procedure, oral or rectal medications would not be optimal. Ketorolac is the NSAID that can be used parenterally (Marino, p. 128).

8. **(c)** Decreased gastrointestinal motility is a common complication of narcotic use. Treatment options should not only include cathartic agents but a reduction in narcotic use, particularly if the patient's pain is well controlled (McPhee, p. 24).

9. **(b)** Deconditioning of the cardiovascular system can occur within days of bedrest. To avoid this process, avoid bedrest if possible. If it is not possible to avoid bedrest, the patient should be positioned as close to upright as possible several times a day in order to decrease cardiovascular deconditioning. Although sitting the patient on the side of the bed may be helpful, it will not help in maintaining cardiovascular integrity (Resnick, p. 54).

10. **(a)** A thromboembolism of the lower extremity may present with slight swelling of the affected calf. A duplex ultrasound of the lower extremity is non-invasive and should detect thrombus in the larger veins (Tierney & Messina, pp. 467-468).

11. **(c)** Coagulopathy is a secondary risk factor for the development of DVT. It should be remembered that although a patient may have a coagulopathy, prophylaxis for DVT still needs to be ordered. Although obesity is a risk factor for DVT, an increased BSA does not indicate obesity (Whelan, p. 20).

12. **(b)** The main causes for immobility in the elderly include weakness, stiffness, pain, imbalance, or psychiatric problems. Because of the patient's recent loss, depression is a very strong possibility and an assessment for depression should be done (Resnick, pp. 53-54).

References

Goodenberg, D. (1998). Medical emergencies. In L. M. Tierney, Jr., S. J. McPhee, & M. A. Papadakis (Eds.), *Current medical diagnosis and treatment* (37th ed., pp. 494-526). Stamford, CT: Appleton & Lange.

Marino, P. L. (1998). *The ICU Book* (2nd ed.). Baltimore: Williams & Wilkins.

McPhee, S. J., & Schroeder, S. A. (1998). In L. M. Tierney, Jr., S. J. McPhee, & M. A. Papadakis (Eds.), *Current medical diagnosis and treatment* (37th ed., pp. 1-30). Stamford, CT: Appleton & Lange.

Resnick, N. M. (1998). Geriatric medicine. In L. M. Tierney, Jr., S. J. McPhee, & M. A. Papadakis (Eds.), *Current medical diagnosis and treatment* (37th ed., pp. 43-64). Stamford, CT: Appleton & Lange.

Tierney, Jr., L. M., & Messina, L. M. (1998). Blood vessels and lymphatics. In L. M. Tierney, Jr., S. J. McPhee, & M. A. Papadakis (Eds.), *Current medical diagnosis and treatment* (37th ed., pp. 448-478). Stamford, CT: Appleton & Lange.

Whelan, A. J., & Mutha, S. (1998). Patient care in internal medicine. In C. F. Carey, H. H. Lee, & K. F. Woeltje (Eds.), *The Washington manual of medical therapeutics* (29th ed., pp. 1-25). Philadelphia: Lippincott-Raven.

Patient Education and Nutrition

Lynn A. Kelso

Select one best answer to the following questions.

1. A 46-year-old female was involved in a motor vehicle accident 12 hours ago. She sustained a head injury and has not yet regained consciousness. Her family has discussed her living will and wants to limit care after 24 hours. You explain that:
    a. Only a durable power of attorney can enforce the living will
    b. It is too early to know if her injuries will be permanent or fatal
    c. The living will is only valid when signed by both patient and family
    d. You will uphold the family's wishes and limit care in 24 hours

2. You are caring for a 59-year-old male who suffered an acute myocardial infarction (MI) five days ago. The patient and his wife have been reading literature, and they understand about diet and exercise, but they are concerned about his ability to return to work. The ACNP should educate them about the use of:
    a. An echocardiogram
    b. A coronary arteriogram
    c. Exercise testing
    d. Cardiac rehabilitation

3. A 63-year-old patient newly diagnosed with diabetes is admitted through the emergency department for hypoglycemia. He was well controlled when discharged from the hospital three days ago. The appropriate intervention would be to:
    a. Discontinue his insulin and begin an oral hypoglycemic agent
    b. Have the patient show you how he draws up his insulin
    c. Order a 24 hour diet and exercise recall
    d. Order blood, urine, and sputum cultures to rule out infection

4. You are reviewing the home plan of care for a 22-year-old patient with moder-

ate asthma. She is able to use her peak flow meter without difficulty, and states that if it is 50% of her personal best she would alter her medication and seek medical attention. You tell her that she:

    a. Is following the appropriate plan of care
    b. Should alter her medication at 80% of personal best
    c. Does not need to seek medical attention at 50% of personal best
    d. Should contact her physician at 80% of personal best

5. While providing a patient with total enteral nutrition, the laboratory test which will best show the patient's response to nutritional therapy is:

    a. Serum albumin
    b. Serum transferrin
    c. Nitrogen balance
    d. Total protein

6. A 21-year-old female being treated for anorexia nervosa is admitted to your service with a syncopal episode. Her laboratory work is significant for a glucose of 51 mg/dL, Na^+ 152 mEq/L, and phosphorus 2.8 mEq/L. The appropriate interventions include correcting her electrolytes and:

    a. Increasing her caloric intake
    b. Decreasing her caloric intake
    c. Beginning potassium phosphate and sodium phosphate 1 pkg t.i.d.
    d. Changing enteral feeds to high protein formula

7. A patient is started on enteral feedings 24 hours after being admitted following MVA. Within 12 hours the patient has 425 cc of loose stool. The appropriate action would be to:

    a. Order *Clostridium difficile* cultures
    b. Begin metronidazole 500 mg p.o. t.i.d.
    c. Change to parenteral nutrition
    d. Decrease enteral feedings

8. A patient who is being dialyzed for acute renal failure following a 35% full-thickness burn injury is on total enteral nutrition. Morning laboratory studies reveal Na^+ 142 mEq/L, K^+ 5.3 mEq/L, BUN 93 mg/dL, and creatinine 2.1 mg/dL. She has been dialyzed daily with minimal decrease in her BUN. The appropriate action would be to:

    a. Continue to dialyze daily for elevated BUN

b. Decrease protein intake due to the increased BUN
c. Place on continuous renal replacement therapy
d. Change to total parenteral nutrition

9. A 29-year-old male with a long standing history of colon cancer and short gut syndrome is on total parenteral nutrition at home. He is admitted to the hospital for evaluation of increasing somnolence and disorientation. Initial orders should include:

a. A lipid profile
b. A head CT scan
c. Liver function studies
d. A lumbar puncture

10. You are calculating nutritional requirements for a 92 kg female whose admitting dry weight was 75 kg. The patient will require total parenteral nutrition due to continued GI bleeding and loss of gut integrity. Along with 500 mL of 20% lipid emulsion, your orders include:

a. 1000 mL; 15% dextrose; 4% AA
b. 1500 mL; 20% dextrose; 6% AA
c. 2000 mL; 25% dextrose; 8% AA
d. 2500 mL; 20% dextrose; 5% AA

11. When assessing the nutritional status of a patient it is important to include:

a. Morning weight
b. 24 hour calorie count
c. Diet record
d. Nitrogen balance

12. A 28-year-old trauma victim had a duodenal feeding tube placed endoscopically. He is currently on full enteral tube feedings at 70 cc per hour. The nurse caring for him informs you that his residual was 140 cc. An abdominal film shows the tip of the feeding tube in the 3rd portion of the duodenum (D-3). The most appropriate response is to:

a. Hold tube feedings for one hour and reassess
b. Continue tube feedings as ordered
c. Discontinue tube feedings
d. Hold tube feedings for four hours and restart at lower rate

Answers and Rationale

1. **(b)** A living will is only applicable when the patient is unable to make decisions for herself and is in a terminal condition. At this time it is too early to know if the patient is in a terminal state, and so the advanced directives are not applicable at this time (Levy, p. 26).

2. **(c)** Before hospital discharge, or within a few days of discharge, patients with a recent acute MI should undergo exercise testing to assess functional ability to perform functions both at home and work. Stress testing will also enable the practitioner to evaluate the patient's current medical regime (Ryan, p. 2343).

3. **(c)** It is important to evaluate for factors that would have decreased this patient's need for exogenous insulin, such as decreased food intake or activity. It is not appropriate to discontinue insulin based upon one episode of hypoglycemia, and screening for infection is not necessary as infection would raise rather than lower serum blood sugar. As this patient was just discharged and well controlled three days ago, the ACNP would reasonably assume that he can draw his insulin correctly, although if the diet and exercise recall is noncontributory it would then be appropriate to observe his technique (Karam, p. 1115).

4. **(b)** The NIH guidelines recommend that moderate to severe asthmatics should alter their regime at 80% of their personal best on the peak flow meter. If they reach 50% or less of their personal best they are having severe asthma symptoms. The altered medical regime should be planned by the patient and the practitioner and must be individualized for each patient, but it should be clearly written in the patient's home plan of care (NIH guidelines, p. 16).

5. **(c)** Circulating protiens are of limited value when assessing the response to nutritional support. These values will change with fluctuations in total body water. Nitrogen balance is the best option in order to assess a response to nutritional support. A 24 hour urine is required to measure urinary urea nitrogen (UUN). Nitrogen balance can then be calculated: Nitrogen balance = (24 hour protein intake/6.25) - ([UUN/0.8] + 2) The goal is to achieve a positive balance (Chan, p. 36).

6. **(b)** Refeeding syndrome occurs in severely malnourished individuals who are being treated with high carbohydrate feedings. These feedings cause an increase in insulin secretion which leads to a cellular uptake of glucose and phosphorus. Severe hypoglycemia and hypophosphatemia can be life threatening if not treated. While correcting fluid and electrolyte disturbances, calories should be cut back to match metabolic demands while replenishing protein. This can then slowly be advanced as tolerated (Chan, p. 38).

7. **(d)** Diarrhea is the most common complication of enteral feeding. When diarrhea is closely associated with the start of enteral feedings, the easiest way to determine cause is to drop the feedings to a trophic level and then slowly advance to goal rate. If a hyperosmolar enteral solution is being used, the strength should be reduced and then slowly advanced as tolerated. If this does not stop the diarrhea, additional studies may be needed (Baron, p. 1177).

8. **(a)** In patients with high protein requirements, such as those with burn injuries, you are unable to decrease protein intake because of rising BUN levels. The only course of action is to continue to dialyze the patient according to BUN level (Cohen, p. 1455).

9. **(c)** Hepatic dysfunction is common in patients on long term parenteral nutrition. This patient has evidence of encephalopathy and liver function should be assessed (Chan, p. 35).

10. **(a)** Without direct or indirect calorimetry to know what the patient's caloric requirements are, it is generally accepted to use 30 to 35 kcal/kg as total caloric requirements. Protein requirements are met with 1.2 to 1.5 gm/kg. Nutritional requirements should be based upon dry weight. This formula will provide the patient with 90 g of protein and 2020 nonprotein calories. The use of protein calories for energy expenditure remains controversial (Chan, pp. 26-28).

11. **(c)** Nutritional risk factors should be addressed in the history and physical examination. The best way to begin to assess nutritional status is to do a dietary record or a 24 hour dietary recall (Baron, p. 1156).

12. **(b)** When the feeding tube is positioned beyond the pylorus, residual counts are not accurate. Duodenal secretions account for a portion of the drainage being measured and should not be considered part of the tube feeding residual. The liver produces and secretes 600 to 1200 mL of bile per day while the gallbladder can store only 100 to 150 mL of bile. The duodenum has many secretions including mucus, enterogastrone, secretin, and cholecystokinin (Matassarin-Jacobs, pp. 1691, 1835).

References

Baron, R. B. (1998). Nutrition. In L. M. Tierney, Jr., S. J. McPhee, & M. A. Papadakis (Eds.), *Current medical diagnosis and treatment* (37th ed., pp. 1150-1179). Stamford, CT: Appleton & Lange.

Chan, M. F. (1998). Nutritional therapy. In C. F. Carey, H. H. Lee, & K. F. Woeltje (Eds.), *The Washington manual of medical therapeutics* (29th ed., pp. 26-38). Philadelphia: Lippincott-Raven.

Cohen, R., & Moelleken, B. R. W. (1998). Disorders due to physical agents. In L. M. Tierney, Jr., S. J. McPhee, & M. A. Papadakis (Eds.), *Current medical diagnosis and treatment* (37th ed., pp. 1443-1464). Stamford, CT: Appleton & Lange.

Highlights of the expert panel report #2. *Guidelines for the diagnosis and management of asthma.* (1997). National Institutes of Health/National Heart, Lung, and Blood Institute. Publication #97-4051a.

Karam, J. H. (1998). Diabetes mellitus and hypoglycemia. In L. M. Tierney, Jr., S. J. McPhee, & M. A. Papadakis (Eds.), *Current medical diagnosis and treatment* (37th ed., pp. 1095-1137). Stamford, CT: Appleton & Lange.

Levy, S. A. (1996). Advanced directives. In R. E. Rakel, & R. M. Kleberg, (Eds.), *Saunders manual of medical practice.* Philadelphia: W. B. Saunders.

Matassarin-Jacobs, E. (1997). Structure and function of the gastrointestinal system. In J. M. Black, & E. Matassarin-Jacobs (Eds.), *Medical-surgical nursing: Clinical management for continuity of care* (5th ed., pp. 1685-1697). Philadelphia: W. B. Saunders.

Matassarin-Jacobs, E. (1997). Structure and function of the liver, biliary tract, and exocrine pancreas. In J. M. Black, & E. Matassarin-Jacobs (Eds.), *Medical-surgical nursing: Clinical management for continuity of care* (5th ed., pp. 1835-1842). Philadelphia: W. B. Saunders.

Psychosocial Issues

Candis Morrison
Lynn A. Kelso

Select one best answer to the following questions.

Questions 1 and 2 refer to the following scenario.

R. S. is a 57-year-old widow of six years. Over the course of the past two years she has experienced intermittent episodes of anorexia, difficulty sleeping, fatigue, and lethargy. She has to force herself to leave the house to participate in activities that she formerly enjoyed. She has a negative past medical and surgical history with the exception of a total abdominal hysterectomy 14 years ago for fibroids. The physical examination does not reveal any abnormalities.

1. The most likely diagnosis for this patient is:

   a. Bipolar disorder
   b. Adjustment disorder
   c. Agoraphobia
   d. Major depression

2. To differentiate between the suspected diagnosis and a normal grief reaction, The ACNP considers the:

   a. Duration of the symptoms
   b. Severity of the symptoms
   c. Associated vegetative symptoms
   d. History of loss of her spouse

3. A 19-year-old female is brought to the urgent care center by her mother. The mother describes a behavior change in her daughter after she attended a party three days ago. Drug abuse is suspected and a urine toxicology screen was ordered during triage. Urine toxicology screens are reliable for detecting which substance up to three days following ingestion?

     a. Barbiturates
     b. Alcohol
     c. Stimulants
     d. Opioids

4. A 19-year-old male comes to the urgent care center requesting a HIV test. Night sweats and palpitations have been waking him from sleep for the past 10 days. He heard on a radio talk show that these symptoms could be connected with AIDS. His social history is negative for high risk sexual behaviors or substance use. On further questioning he reports that he is failing calculus and physics and has not informed his parents. If his grade point average does not improve he will have to leave school. He recently lost his part time job and he is unable to make his car payment. The ACNP suspects that he is suffering from:

     a. HIV/AIDS
     b. Anxiety
     c. Dysthymic disorder
     d. Tuberculosis

5. You are the ACNP caring for an alcoholic gentlemen post coronary artery bypass graft. He is preparing for discharge and expresses a need for help with his drinking problem. One of the most effective treatments for alcoholism is:

     a. Antidepressant medication
     b. Aversion therapy with disulfiram
     c. Anxiolytics
     d. Active participation in Alcoholics Anonymous

6. W.A., a 32-year-old female, is brought to the emergency department with a fractured right radius and facial ecchymoses. The ACNP notes that her story of the mechanism of injury is not consistent with objective findings. Her records reveal that she has had multiple injuries treated over the past three years. Historical factors which may lead you to suspect domestic violence include:

     a. A history of substance abuse in her spouse
     b. A spouse > 40 years old
     c. A partner of minority cultural background
     d. A household income < $25,000.00 per year

7. A 73-year-old male is newly diagnosed with Alzheimer's disease. He currently needs assistance with ADL and has been found wandering the halls of the hospital. His 70-ycar-old wife is to be his primary caregiver. When assessing her

ability to cope with this burden the ACNP knows that the factor that would put her at greatest risk for negative consequences of caregiving is:

    a. History as a victim of a crime
    b. The fact that she lives with the care receiver
    c. A lack of activities outside the home
    d. The severity of the care receiver's symptoms

8. A 48-year-old female being treated for ovarian cancer is being seen by you for the first time. During the interview you discover that she is married with a 14-year-old daughter living at home. Although she is no longer able to work and has recently been unable to keep up with housework, her husband has a good job that requires travel and her daughter has been helping around the house. She has been feeling depressed since her activity decreased. While discussing her depression, you ask about:

    a. Anger she has toward her husband
    b. Guilt she has related to her daughter
    c. Fear about her future
    d. Denial of her disease process

9. A 42-year-old female has metastatic breast cancer. She remains comfortable on a continuous MSO_4 infusion and is able to minimally participate in ADL. Her husband is her primary caregiver and he comes to you to discuss a code status for his wife. With respect to the ethical principles that guide nursing practice, the one that takes priority when there is conflict is:

    a. Autonomy
    b. Beneficence
    c. Fidelity
    d. Justice

10. You are evaluating a 71-year-old male who suffered a brain attack three years ago. Although he is functional with minimal assistance at home, he has recently become incontinent of urine. His wife is his primary caregiver, and she is concerned about this development and is frustrated with not being able to do anything to help. You then discuss with them:

    a. A caregiver support group
    b. Incontinence aids available
    c. A continence program
    d. Stress reduction techniques

Answers and Rationale

1. **(d)** One can make a diagnosis of major depression if five of the nine major depression symptoms are present: Depressed mood, anhedonia (lack of interest or pleasure in all or almost all activities), sleep disorder, appetite change, fatigue or loss of energy, psychomotor retardation or agitation, trouble concentrating or difficulty making decisions, low self-esteem or guilt, recurrent thoughts of death, or suicidal ideation (Cole, p. 1739).

2. **(a)** DSM-IV indicates that if depressive symptoms are still present two months following the loss, the diagnosis of major depressive disorder may be made (Cole, p. 1739).

3. **(a)** The usefulness of urine toxicology screening for detection of drugs varies markedly, primarily determined by the pharmacokinetics of the drugs. Water soluble drugs (alcohol, stimulants, opioids) are eliminated in approximately 24 hours. Barbiturates and tetrahydrocannabinol persist for several days (Eisendrath, p. 1000).

4. **(b)** Generalized anxiety disorder is the most common anxiety disorder. It appears between 20 and 35 years of age. The disabling anxiety symptoms of apprehension, worry, irritability, hypervigilance, and somatic complaints are present for more than one month. Tachycardia, increased BP, epigastric distress, headache, and syncope are common symptoms. Some of the origins or exacerbating causes can be identified in life situations (Eisendrath, p. 978).

5. **(d)** Successful abstinence is proportionate to the utilization of Alcoholics Anonymous (Eisendrath, p. 1017).

6. **(a)** This is a typical history of a battered woman. Though no well defined criteria exist to predict who will be battered, factors have identified some high risk characteristics: (a) Those who are single, divorced, or planning a separation, (b) those between the ages of 17 and 28, (c) those who abuse alcohol or other drugs or whose partners do, (d) those who are pregnant and (e) those whose partners are excessively jealous or possessive. There are no economic or racial predictors of women at risk (McHugh & Salasar, p. 1676).

7. **(b)** Although there are a variety of factors that are felt to contribute to the negative consequences of caregiving, the living arrangement is felt to be the most powerful determinant. Caregivers who reside in the same household as care receivers report more negative physical, emotional, and social consequences, regardless of relationship, and controlling for a variety of other factors (Bass & Noelker, p. 254).

8. **(b)** Although there is little research on young caregivers of ill adults, the literature does show that parents feel guilty about young or adolescent children becoming their caregivers. Since her depression began at about the time the daughter had to increase her role as caregiver, this is a good area upon which to focus (Gates, p. 12).

9. **(a)** When discussing life sustaining treatment decisions, the ethical principles that guide nursing practice should be followed. When ethical principles conflict autonomy (the competent patient's right to make decisions regarding care) should prevail (Ouslander, et al., p. 444).

10. **(c)** Both the patient and the caregiver may well benefit from a continence program which can be devised by the practitioner to assist with specific urinary incontinence problems affecting this patient. This may include such things as bladder retraining and habit training (Beheshti & Fonteyn, p. 392).

References

Bass, D. M., & Noelker, L. S. (1997). Family caregiving: A focus for aging research and intervention. In K. F. Ferraro (Ed.), *Gerontology perspectives and issues* (2nd ed., pp. 243-264). New York: Springer.

Beheshti, P., & Fonteyn, M. (1998). Role of the advanced practice nurse in continence care in the home. *AACN Clinical Issues: Advanced Practice in Acute and Critical Care, 9*(2), 389-395.

Cole, S. A. (1996). Mood disorders. In J. Noble (Ed.), *Textbook of primary care medicine* (2nd ed.). St. Louis: Mosby.

Eisendrath, S. J. (1998). Psychiatric disorders. In L. M. Tierney, Jr., S. J. McPhee, & M. A. Papadakis (Eds.), *Current medical diagnosis and treatment* (37th ed.). Stamford, CT: Appleton & Lange.

Gates, M. F., & Lackey, N. R. (1998). Youngsters caring for adults with cancer. *Image: Journal of nursing scholarship, 30*(1), 11-15.

McHugh, M., Salasar, C. M., & Rich, J. A. (1996). Domestic violence. In J. Noble (Ed.), *Textbook of primary care medicine* (2nd ed.). St. Louis: Mosby.

Ouslander, J. G., Osterweil, D., & Morley, J. (1997). *Medical care in the nursing home.* NY: McGraw-Hill.

Professional Issues and Trends in Advanced Practice

Ruth M. Kleinpell

Select one best answer to the following questions.

1. An ACNP is seeking certification after graduating from a master's level ACNP program. Which of the following is true about certification?

    a. It is required by all States for practice as an ACNP
    b. It authorizes the ACNP to perform indicated tests and treatments in the care of the acutely ill patient
    c. It is a State recognized mechanism to ensure competency
    d. It establishes that the ACNP has met certain standards and skill mastery in the care of acutely ill patients

2. When on a job interview, the ACNP is asked to describe her scope of practice. Which of the following best describes the scope of practice for the ACNP?

    a. It is directed toward managing acute and critically ill patients primarily in ICU settings
    b. It includes restorative and rehabilitative aspects of patient care
    c. It is team oriented and focuses on direct patient care management
    d. It is collaborative but requires physician supervision for invasive skills

3. While interviewing for a hospital based position, the ACNP is told that the job description includes research. Which of the following statements is not true regarding the ACNP's role in research?

    a. It is primarily involved in assisting with data collection
    b. It involves identifying potential research problems
    c. It is limited as patient care concerns are a priority
    d. It does not involve the process of research utilization

4. The monitoring of outcomes is important in establishing the effectiveness of the ACNP role. The focus of outcomes assessment for the ACNP should:

   a. Emphasize tracking survival, length of stay, and costs of treatment
   b. Compare nurse practitioner care to physician care to establish the effectiveness of the role
   c. Include both performance appraisal and patient outcomes of care
   d. Analyze complications which occur during treatment

5. The ACNP is now eligible for Medicare reimbursement. Reimbursement of NP services to Medicare patients:

   a. Can vary from State to State
   b. Consists of part A covering outpatient care and part B covering inpatient care
   c. Requires the NP to work in collaboration with a physician in some States
   d. Allows direct NP reimbursement in some settings

6. Which of the following is correct regarding prescriptive privileges for the ACNP?

   a. They are granted after educational requirements are completed and national certification has been obtained
   b. They are obtained through contractual agreements with physician practice groups or hospital medical board credentialing
   c. They are granted based on State practice acts and may restrict the prescription of controlled substances
   d. They are dependent on individual State nurse practice acts and employment arrangements

7. Sally T. has been hired as an ACNP to work with a group of cardiologists. Her role will incorporate both inpatient care and outpatient clinic responsibilities. Her ACNP position:

   a. Will require her to obtain credentialing privileges for hospital practice
   b. Will encompass substitutive care traditionally given by physicians
   c. Is considered to be a service based practice model
   d. Must be supervised by a physician in the inpatient setting

8. Which of the following statements is not characteristic of the standards of professional performance for the ACNP?

   a. The ACNP participates in quality monitoring
   b. The ACNP uses organizational resources in caring for the patient

    c. The ACNP evaluates clinical practice in relation to professional practice standards

    d. The ACNP subscribes to a professional malpractice insurance policy

9. Which of the following is correct regarding graduate education in nursing?

    a. All programs are accredited by the JCAHO

    b. All programs are accredited by the AACN

    c. It is required for nurse practitioners in all States

    d. It is required for obtaining prescriptive privileges in some States

10. Malpractice insurance can be divided into two types—claims based and occurrence based. Occurrence based malpractice insurance:

    a. Protects against any incidents occurring during the time the policy was in effect

    b. Protects against any incidents that occurred during the period of the contract

    c. Protects against any occurrence regardless of the practice setting

    d. Protects against any incident as long as the policy is current

11. Legal regulation of advanced nursing practice:

    a. Is the responsibility of the American Nurses Association

    b. Is the responsibility of the State board of nursing

    c. Is the joint responsibility of State legislators and boards of nursing

    d. Falls under the jurisdiction of State boards of medicine

12. Various mechanisms can influence the practice of nursing. The most restrictive level of regulation in nursing practice is:

    a. Credentialing

    b. Registration

    c. Certification

    d. Licensure

13. Certification is acknowledged as being essential for advanced practice nurses. A criticism of certification in advanced practice nursing is that:

    a. Uniform standards between types of certification is lacking

    b. National certification does not confer prescriptive authority

    c. Requirements for certification can vary between States

    d. State practice acts designate the type of credentialing recognized in a State

14. An ACNP is working in collaborative practice and is seeking clinical privileges. Clinical privileges for the ACNP:

    a. Are granted with successful completion of national ACNP certification
    b. Are institution based
    c. Are regulated by the State board of medicine
    d. Are required for hospital based practice

15. Nurse T., an ACNP, is authorized to dispense medications according to a State regulating board approved list of prescription drugs. This is an example of which type of prescriptive authority:

    a. State statute prescriptive authority
    b. Collaborative arrangement prescriptive authority
    c. Formulary prescriptive authority
    d. Controlled substance prescriptive authority

16. An ACNP is asked to consult on a complex acutely ill patient for wound care management. Which of the following is not a component of the role of the ACNP as consultant/collaborator?

    a. Patient advocate
    b. Information expert
    c. Formal consultation
    d. Implementing care protocols

17. Research can be categorized as experimental and nonexperimental. Nonexperimental research:

    a. Is the strongest type of research design for a study
    b. Involves manipulation of variables but lacks a control group
    c. Describes or examines relationships among variables
    d. Tests the effects of an intervention or experiment

18. Which of the following steps is not included in the research process?

    a. Review related literature
    b. Choose a research design
    c. Seek funding for analysis
    d. Interpret the results

19. Health care is a recognized priority of health policy and legislation. Which of the following is not included in the Healthy People 2000 goal statement?

   a. Preventing disease transmission
   b. Achieving access to health prevention services
   c. Reducing health disparities
   d. Increasing the span of healthy life

20. Performance of a routine Pap smear is considered which level of health prevention?

   a. Primary
   b. Secondary
   c. Tertiary
   d. Rehabilitative

21. Mrs. W. is a 75-year-old patient who suffered a cerebral infarct two weeks ago. After a turbulent hospital course, she is finally ready for discharge. The ACNP has referred Mrs. W. to an inpatient rehabilitation facility. This is an example of which level of health prevention?

   a. Primary
   b. Secondary
   c. Tertiary
   d. Rehabilitative

22. Medicare and Medicaid provide coverage for health care services. Which of the following is true with regard to Medicaid?

   a. It is a federally funded and administered health program
   b. It is a State funded and administered health program
   c. It is a government sponsored supplemental medical insurance
   d. It is a federally supported, State administered health program

23. The Patient Self-Determination Act of 1990 requires that all patients have the right to:

   a. Make an advanced directive
   b. Designate a legal guardian
   c. Designate a power of attorney
   d. Designate end of life care choices

24. The ACNP is asked to determine if a newly admitted patient can give consent to an invasive procedure. In order to give informed consent, the patient must not necessarily be able to:

   a. Make decisions about his care

b. Understand and reason
c. Repeat explanations about their care
d. Communicate and reason

25. The ethical principle of fidelity is the duty to:

    a. Be fair
    b. Be truthful
    c. Do no harm
    d. Be faithful

26. Monitoring of outcomes is important for ACNP practice. Which of the following is not included in the outcomes of care?

    a. Rehospitalization rates
    b. Adverse events
    c. Long term results of treatment
    d. Managing complications

27. Nurse H., an ACNP, is responsible for monitoring quality initiatives in the critical care area. Part of one initiative is to monitor the qualifications of the nursing staff. This is an example of monitoring:

    a. Processes of care
    b. Outcomes of care
    c. Structures of care
    d. Resources of care

28. Continuous qualilty improvement is used to assess health care providers' and health care agencies' performance. Which of the following is not a component of quality assurance?

    a. Monitoring care quality
    b. Monitoring cost of care
    c. Peer review
    d. Monitoring patient satisfaction

29. The ACNP is a member of a committee working on a quality improvement initiative to better structure care after open heart surgery, including when vital signs, laboratory and diagnostic tests, and aspects of care are to be completed. This is an example of:

    a. Quality planning
    b. Diagnosis related group (DRG) care

  c. Developing a critical pathway

  d. Multidisciplinary care

30. Various mechanisms can influence the regulation of advanced practice nursing. Which of the following is not included in the regulation of advanced practice nursing?

  a. State nurse practice acts

  b. Certification

  c. Peer review

  d. Institutional practice privileging

31. An ACNP is relocating and seeking licensure to practice in a new State of residence. Licensure is granted by:

  a. An agency of State government

  b. A voluntary nongovernmental agency

  c. A national governmental agency

  d. A State nongovernmental agency

32. A newly hired ACNP negotiates for malpractice insurance coverage as part of her employment benefits. Malpractice insurance:

  a. Will protect the ACNP from charges related to invasive procedural work traditionally performed by a physician

  b. Will only protect the ACNP from charges related to injury to the patient

  c. Will not protect the ACNP from charges of practicing medicine without a license if practicing outside the legal scope of practice for the state

  d. Will protect the ACNP from charges of practicing medicine without a license as long as clinical privilege have been obtained

33. Medicare health coverage is divided into parts A and B. Medicare part B covers:

  a. Short term skilled nursing facility care

  b. Hospice care

  c. Home health agency visits

  d. Outpatient hospital care

34. An ACNP is employed by a managed care network to practice in a multipractice clinic. Which of the following is accurate regarding managed care networks?

  a. They contractually agree to provide services for certain patient groups

b. They usually allow the patient to choose a provider, but not a hospital
c. They are funded with a fixed percentage of federal dollars
d. They provide reimbursement to nurse practitioners through provider arrangements

35. For Medicare reimbursement, services of nurse practitioners performed "incident-to" physician services means:

    a. The physician was unavailable to perform the service
    b. The nurse practitioner performed the service with direct supervision of the physician
    c. The nurse practitioner performed services ordinarily performed by the physician
    d. The nurse practitioner performed the service without the physician being present

36. Nurse practitioners can be reimbursed nationally through which of the following?

    a. CHAMPUS
    b. Private insurance companies
    c. Managed care networks
    d. Social Security Administration

37. Preferred Provider Organizations (PPO) are:

    a. A fee-for-service provider partnership
    b. A type of HMO
    c. A type of managed care system
    d. An HMO subplan

38. Which of the following is accurate regarding the National Practitioner Data Bank?

    a. It is a professional registry for advanced practice nurses
    b. It is a governmental resource of current legislation pertinent to nurse practitioner practice
    c. It provides voluntary listings for physicians and advanced practice nurses by professional area of expertise
    d. It compiles information on medical-legal actions taken against health care professionals

Answers and Rationale

1. **(d)** Certification establishes that a person has met certain standards in a particular profession which signifies mastery of specialized knowledge and skills. Certification is granted by nongovernmental agencies such as specialty boards and nationally by the American Nurses Credentialing Center. Individual state practice acts designate if certification is required for ACNP practice (Porscher, pp. 182-186).

2. **(b)** The scope of practice of an ACNP is broad based, with the focus of care being restorative, rehabilitative or maintenance of new, chronic, or terminal illnesses. The ACNP practices in a variety of settings, including tertiary and secondary health care centers. The practice setting will dictate components of the role and the degree of supervision required for various responsibilities (American Nurses Association, 1995, pp. 11-13).

3. **(b)** The ACNP's role in research includes participation in all phases of the research process, research evaluation and critique, research utilization, and research dissemination. There is no greater emphasis on any specific part of the process, and should not be limited in one or all aspects in favor of patient care (American Nurses Association, 1995, pp. 28-29).

4. **(c)** Assessing and monitoring the outcome of ACNP care is important in establishing role effectiveness. Outcome assessment for the ACNP should include both performance appraisal (evaluation of ACNP performance) and patient outcomes of care. Option "a" does not include performance appraisal, option "b" is incorrect as ACNP outcome assessment does not include comparison to other care providers, and option "d" does not reflect outcomes at all (American Nurses Association, 1995, pp. 24-25).

5. **(c)** Medicare is a federally funded health program with part A covering inpatient hospital and post hospital skilled nursing care, home health, and hospice. Part B is a supplemental medical insurance which covers physician visits, outpatient care, home care, laboratory, radiology and other related medical services and supplies. Direct Medicare reimbursement can be obtained for NP services provided in both rural and urban settings at 85% of physician reimbursement for services provided in collaboration with a physician (McCarthy & Berman, p. 73).

6. **(c)** The ability of the ACNP to prescribe medications to clients is dependent on State nursing practice acts. Prescriptive authority varies in terms of the type of physician supervision or collaboration required and whether controlled substances are included in prescription writing/dispensing authority (Pearson, pp. 14-16, 19-20).

7. **(c)** ACNP practice models include service based, practice based, and population based practice models. Service based ACNP are involved with clinical management of specific patients followed by a medical or surgical group such as surgical oncology or neurology. Practice based ACNPs are involved with clinical management of patients seen on a particular hospital unit or clinic setting, such as vascular surgery patients. Population based ACNP are involved with patients with specific disease entities, such as diabetes. Hospital credentialing and privileging may be required for ACNP practice in the hospital setting. Those privileges would also stipulate the degree of direct supervision required. ACNP practice is not substitutive for physician care, but rather is a comprehensive collaborative care model (Kleinpell, 1998, p. 158).

8. **(d)** As a component of the standards of clinical practice for the acute care nurse practitioner, the standards of professional performance describe a competent level of behavior in the professional role including activities related to quality of care, performance appraisal, education, collegiality, ethics, collaboration, research, and resource utilization. Subscribing to a professional malpractice insurance policy is not included in these specific standards and is optional for advanced practice nurses (American Nurses Association, 1995, p. 23).

9. **(d)** The JCAHO does not accredit graduate programs in nursing. Graduate education programs in nursing may be accredited by the AACN, but many are not. Some programs are accredited by the NLN, and others are not accredited at all. Although most nurse practitioner programs in existence at this time are graduate programs, many nurse practitioners practicing today were educated in certificate programs and are presently not required to earn a master's degree. Choice ''d'' is a correct statement—some, but not all, States require a master's degree for prescriptive privileges (Pearson, pp. 14-16, 19-20, 25-26, 29-33, 39, 43-46, 49-50, 52-54, 57-58, 61-62, 64, 66).

10. **(a)** Occurrence based malpractice insurance protects against any incident that

occurred during the time the policy was in effect even if the claim is made when the policy is no longer in effect (Busby, pp. 693-694).

11. **(c)** Legal regulation of advanced nursing practice is the joint responsibility of State legislators and boards of nursing (Porcher, p. 179).

12. **(d)** The most restrictive level of regulation in nursing practice is licensure (Porcher, p. 180).

13. **(a)** A criticism of credentialing is that uniform standards between different types of certification is lacking. While national certification is recognized by all States, it may not be a requirement for practice within a state (Stanley & Bednash, pp. 145-147).

14. **(b)** Clinical priviliges for the ACNP are institution based and are usually granted by the medical staff. Practice agreements and protocols with a collaborating physician, along with a written scope of practice are usually required to obtain advanced practice privileges within an institution (Stanley & Bednash, pp. 160-162).

15. **(c)** Dispensing medications according to a State regulated board approved list of prescription drugs is an example of formulary prescriptive authority (American Nurses Association, 1996, pp. 10-12).

16. **(d)** Components of the role of the ACNP as consultant/collaborator include both formal and informal consultation, serving as an information expert, making referrals, and being a patient advocate. Implementing care protocols is a component of the role of the ACNP as clinician (American Nurses Association, 1995, p. 12, 28).

17. **(c)** Nonexperimental research aims to describe situations and experiences or examine relationships among variables (Polit & Hungler, pp. 176-178).

18. **(c)** Steps in the research process include formulating the research problem, reviewing related literature, formulating hypotheses, selecting research design, identifying the population to be studied, specifying methods of data

collection, designing the study, conducting the study, analyzing the data, interpreting the results and communicating the findings (Polit & Hungler, pp. 31-37).

19. **(a)** *Healthy People 2000* goals include increasing the span of healthy life for all Americans, reducing health disparities among Americans, and achieving access to preventive services for all Americans (Venegoni, pp. 83-84).

20. **(b)** Performance of routine Pap smear is considered to be secondary health prevention (Geoppinger, pp. 66-67; Mladenovich, p. 4).

21. **(c)** Stroke rehabilitation is considered to be tertiary health prevention. (Mladenovich, p. 4).

22. **(d)** Medicaid is a federally supported, State administered health program for low income families and individuals (McCarthy & Berman, pp. 73-74).

23. **(a)** The Patient Self-Determination Act of 1990 requires that all patients have the right to execute an advanced directive (Veatch, p. 370).

24. **(c)** Patient competency implies that the patient is able to make decisions about their care, is able to understand, reason, differentiate good and bad, and communicate (Boyd, et al., p. 47-48).

25. **(d)** The ethical principle of fidelity is the duty to be faithful (Boyd, et al., p. 98).

26. **(d)** Outcomes of care include rehospitalization rates, adverse events, short and long term results of treatment, and complications. Managing complications is a process of care (Fowler, et al., pp. 298-302).

27. **(c)** Structures of care are inputs into care such as resources, equipment, or numbers and qualifications of staff (Fowler, et al., pp. 298-302).

28. **(d)** Components of quality assurance include monitoring of care quality, care appropriateness, effectiveness of care, cost of care, self-regulation, and peer

review to ensure compliance to care standards. Monitoring patient satisfaction is an outcome of care (Satinsky, pp. 126-128, 144).

29. **(c)** A critical pathway contains key patient care activities and time for those activities that are needed for a specific case type of diagnosis related group (DRG). Critical pathways are a blueprint for planning and managing care delivered by all disciplines (Wojner, pp. 136-138).

30. **(d)** Regulation of advanced practice nursing is accomplished through statutes, rules and regulations of State nurse practice acts, certification, peer review, and self-regulation (American Nurses Association, 1996, pp. 2-4).

31. **(a)** Licensure is granted by an agency of State government (Porcher, pp. 180-182).

32. **(c)** Malpractice insurance for the ACNP will not protect the ACNP from charges of practicing medicine without a license if practicing outside the legal scope of practice for the state (Busby, p. 693).

33. **(d)** Medicare part B, a supplemental medical insurance, covers outpatient hospital care, physician visits, home care, laboratory, radiology, and other related services (McCarthy & Berman, pp. 73).

34. **(a)** Managed care networks contractually agree to provide services for certain patient groups (Satinsky, pp. 127-129).

35. **(c)** For Medicare reimbursement, services of nurse practitioners performed "incident-to" physician services means that the nurse practitioner was able to perform services ordinarily performed by the physician (Newman, pp. 556-557).

36. **(a)** Nurse practitioners can be reimbursed nationally through CHAMPUS (Civilian Health and Medical Program of the United Services and FEHBP (Federal Employees Health Benefit Program) (Newman, pp. 559-560).

37. **(c)** Preferred provider organizations are a type of managed care system. A partnership is established between a group of "preferred providers" and an insurance company or entity to provide specific medical and hospital care at prearranged costs (Satinsky, pp. 126-128, 144).

38. **(d)** The National Practitioner Data Bank, a federal entity, compiles information on medical-legal actions taken against health care professionals. Conditions that must be reported include malpractice settlements and adverse actions that influence clinical privileges or licensure. Hospitals are required to query the National Practitioner Data Bank when a provider makes an application for staff or clinical privilege appointments and then every two years thereafter (Busby, p. 693).

References

American Nurses Association. (1996). *Scope and standards of advanced practice registered nursing.* Washington, DC: American Nurses Association.

American Nurses Association. (1995). *Standards of clinical practice and scope of practice for the acute care nurse practitioner.* Washington DC: American Nurses Publishing.

Boyd, K., Higgs, R., & Pinching, A. (1997). *The new dictionary of medical ethics.* London: B. M. J. Publishing.

Busby, L. C. (1999). Advanced practice trends/issues and health policy. In V. L. Millonig & S. K. Miller (Eds.), *Adult nurse practitioner certification review guide* (3rd ed. pp. 685-719). Potomac, MD: Health Leadership Associates.

Fowler Byers, J., & Brunnel, M. (1998). Demonstrating the value of the advanced practice nurse: An evaluation model. *AACN Clinical Issues, 9*(2), 296-305.

Goeppinger, J. (1996). Renaissance of primary care: An opportunity for nursing. In J. Hickey, R. Ouimette, & S. Venegoni (Eds.), *Advanced practice nursing—changing roles and clinical applications* (pp. 63-73). Philadelphia: Lippincott-Raven.

Hickey, J. (1996). Reformation of healthcare and implications for advanced nursing practice. In Hickey, J., Ouimette, R., & Venegoni, S. (Eds.), *Advanced Practice Nursing—Changing Roles and Clinical Applications* (pp. 3-21). Philadelphia: Lippincott-Raven.

Hravnak, M., & Baldisseri, M. (1997). Credentialing and privileging: Insight into the process. *AACN Clinical Issues, 8*(1), 108-115.

King, K., Parrinello, K., & Baggs, J. (1996). Collaboration and advanced practice nursing. In J. Hickey, R. Ouimette, & S. Venegoni (Eds.), *Advanced practice nursing—changing roles and clinical applications* (pp. 146-162). Philadelphia: Lippincott-Raven.

Kleinpell R., & Piano, M. (1998). *Practice issues for the acute care nurse practitioner.* NY: Springer.

Kleinpell, R. (1997). Acute care nurse practitioners: Roles and practice profiles. *AACN Clinical Issues Advanced Practice in Acute and Critical Care, 8*(1), 156-162.

McCarthy, M., & Berman, J. (1998). Corporate health and managed competition: Implications for advanced practice nursing in the new American health care system. In C. Sheehy, & M. McCarthy (Eds.), *Advanced Practice Nursing* (pp. 68-87). Philadelphia: F. A. Davis.

Mladenovic, J. (1995). *Primary care secrets.* St. Louis: Mosby.

Newman, D. (1996). Program and practice management for the advanced practice nurse. In A. Hamric, J. Spross, & C. Hanson (Eds.), *Advanced nursing practice—an integrative approach*. Philadelphia: W. B. Saunders.

Pearson, L. (1998). Annual update of how each State stands on legislative issues affecting advanced nursing practice. *The Nurse Practitioner: The American Journal of Primary Health Care, 23*(1), 14-16, 19-20, 25-26, 29-33, 39, 43-46, 49-50, 52-54, 57-58, 61-62, 64, 66.

Polit, D., & Hungler, B. (1995). *Nursing research: Principles and methods*. Philadelphia: J. B. Lippincott.

Porcher, F. (1996). Licensure, certification, and credentialing. In J. Hickey, R. Ouimette, & S. Venegoni (Eds.). *Advanced practice nursing—changing roles and clinical applications* (pp. 179-187). Philadelphia: Lippincott-Raven.

Rowland, H., & Rowland, B. (1996). *The manual of nursing quality assurance*. Gaithersburg, MD: Aspen.

Satinksy, M. (1996). Advanced practice nurse in a managed care environment. In J. Hickey, R. Ouimette, & S. Venegoni (Eds.), *Advanced practice nursing—changing roles and clinical applications* (pp. 126-145). Philadelphia: Lippincott-Raven.

Stanley, J., & Bednash, G. (1998). Formulation and approval of credentialing and clinical privileges. In C. Sheehy & M. McCarthy (Eds.), *Advanced Practice Nursing* (pp. 140-167). Philadelphia: F. A. Davis.

Veatch, R. (1997). *Medical ethics*. Sudbury, MA: Jones & Bartlett.

Venegoni, S. (1996). Changing environment of healthcare. In J. Hickey, R. Ouimette, & S. Venegoni (Eds.), *Advanced practice nursing—changing roles and clinical applications* (pp. 146-162). Philadelphia: Lippincott-Raven.

Wojner, A. (1996). Outcomes management: An interdisciplinary search for best practice. *AACN Clinical Issues, 7*(1), 133-145.

Health Leadership Associates
Nurse Practitioner Continuing Education
Programs

Analysis of the 12-lead ECG

This course is designed for advanced practice nurses. During this 8 hour course you will review cardiac electrophysiology, the cardiac cycle and cardiac muscle function as a basis for 12-lead ECG interpretation; analysis of dysrhythmia, conduction abnormalities, atrial abnormalities, ventricular hypertrophy, axis deviation, myocardial ischemia and myocardial infarction. A one hour practice workshop completes the program. A comprehensive course syllabus is included.

Pharmacology for Nurse Practitioners: A Comprehensive Review and Update

This 30 hour course is designed as a comprehensive presentation and review of pharmacology from the physiologic perspective. In addition to presenting the pharmacokinetics and pharmacodynamics of drugs (indications, contraindications, mechanisms of action, excretion and side effects profile) the corresponding body system physiology will be presented in a format that makes the pharmacology easy to understand and apply in clinical practice. A comprehensive course syllabus is included.

Suturing Review and Practice

This $2\frac{1}{2}$ hour course is designed for nurse practitioners who do not have significant suturing experience. Whether you have been taught but haven't practiced, or have never been taught at all, this program will introduce and reinforce skills that you have not had the opportunity to develop. A brief didactic session on wound assessment and preparation is followed by hands-on instruction and practice of the simple interrupted and vertical mattress techniques.

For information on these and other programs contact:
Health Leadership Associates, Inc.
P.O. Box 59153
Potomac, MD 20859
1-800-435-4775

For information on Certification Review Courses, Home Study Programs and Review Books contact:

Health Leadership Associates, Inc.
Post Office Box 59153
Potomac, Maryland 20859

1-800-435-4775

REVIEW BOOK/AUDIO CASSETTE ORDER FORM
HEALTH LEADERSHIP ASSOCIATES, INC.

PLEASE PRINT OR TYPE

NAME: _____

ADDRESS: Street _____ Apt. # _____ City _____ State _____ Zip Code _____

TELEPHONE: _____ (HOME) _____ (WORK)

Section 1: AUDIO CASSETTES

Professional "live" audio recordings of Review Courses are approximately 15 hours in length unless otherwise noted and include detailed course handouts. Continuing Education contact hours are available for these audio cassette Home Study Programs.

QTY	REVIEW COURSE TITLE	PRICE	
___	Acute Care Nurse Practitioner	$150.00	___
___	Adult Nurse Practitioner	$150.00	___
___	Analysis of the 12-Lead ECG (Available 6/99)	$75.00	___
___	** Childbearing Management	$ 45.00	___
___	Clinical Specialist in Adult Psychiatric and Mental Health Nursing	$150.00	___
___	Family Nurse Practitioner (Consists of ANP, PNP & Childbearing Management Courses)	$330.00	___
___	* Gerontological Nurse	$ 75.00	___
___	Gerontological Nurse Practitioner	$150.00	___
___	Home Health Nurse	$150.00	___
___	Inpatient Obstetric/Maternal Newborn/ Low Risk Neonatal/Perinatal Nurse	$150.00	___
___	Medical-Surgical Nurse	$150.00	___
___	** Menopause Lecture	$ 30.00	___
___	Midwifery Review	$150.00	___
___	* Pediatric Nurse	$ 75.00	___
___	Pediatric Nurse Practitioner	$150.00	___
___	Pharmacology Review and Update (Available 4/99)	$300.00	___
___	* Psychiatric and Mental Health Nurse	$ 75.00	___
___	** Test Taking Strategies and Techniques	$ 20.00	___
___	Women's Health Care Nurse Practitioner	$150.00	___

* 8 Hour Course, ** 2 Hour Course

SUB TOTAL: _____

Maryland Residents add 5% sales tax: _____

CEU FEE ($25/course, except FNP course $35): OPTIONAL

Shipping: 2 Hour Course $ 5.00 _____

All other Courses $10.00 _____

TOTAL: _____

PAYMENT DUE METHOD OF PAYMENT

☐ Check or money order (US funds, payable to Health Leadership Associates, Inc.) A $25 fee will be charged on returned checks.

☐ Purchase Order is attached. P.O. # _____

☐ Please charge my: ☐ MasterCard ☐ Visa ☐ AMEX ☐ Discover

Credit Card# _____ Exp. date _____

Signature _____

Print Name _____

REVIEW GUIDES & AUDIO CASSETTES

1) Section 1 Total $ _____

2) Section 2 Total $ _____

3) Section 3 Total $ _____ (All prices subject to change without notice)

TOTAL PAYMENT DUE $ _____

Section 2: REVIEW BOOKS

QTY	BOOK TITLE	PRICE	
___	Adult Nurse Practitioner Certification Review Guide (third edition)	$ 47.75	___
___	Family Nurse Practitioner Certification Review Guide Set (Includes ANP, PNP, and Women's Health Care NP Guides)	$123.25	___
___	Gerontological Nursing Certification Review Guide for the Generalist, Clinical Specialist, and Nurse Practitioner (revised edition)	$ 47.75	___
___	Pediatric Nurse Practitioner Certification Review Guide (third edition)	$ 47.75	___
___	Psychiatric Certification Review Guide for the Generalist and Clinical Specialist in Adult, Child, and Adolescent Psychiatric and Mental Health Nursing (second edition)	$ 47.75	___
___	Women's Health Care Nurse Practitioner Certification Review Guide	$ 47.75	___
___	TODAY and TOMORROW'S WOMAN – MENOPAUSE: BEFORE AND AFTER (Girls of 16 to Women of 99)	$ 10.00	___

STUDY QUESTION BOOKS

QTY		PRICE	
___	Acute Care Nurse Practitioner Certification Study Question Book	$ 30.00	___
___	Adult Nurse Practitioner Certification Study Question Book	$ 30.00	___
___	Family Nurse Practitioner Certification Study Question Book Set (Includes ANP, PNP and WHCNP Study Question Books)	$ 60.00	___
___	Pediatric Nurse Practitioner Certification Study Question Book	$ 30.00	___
___	Women's Health Nurse Practitioner Certification Study Question Book	$ 30.00	___

SUB TOTAL: _____

Maryland Residents add 5% sales tax: _____

CEU FEE ($20 per book, except FNP Set $35): OPTIONAL

Shipping: $9.00 FNP Set: _____

$5.00 for one book: _____

$2.00 for each additional book: _____
(Except $1.00 for each add'l. *Today and Tomorrow's Woman*)

TOTAL: _____

For orders of 10 or greater call 1-800-435-4775.

Section 3: REVIEW BOOK/AUDIO CASSETTE DISCOUNT PACKAGES

A discounted rate is available when purchasing Review Book(s) and Audio Cassettes together. When purchasing packages, indicate Book/Audio Cassette selections in sections 1 and 2. *Does not apply to Study Question Books.* Calculate amount due in this section.

QTY	PACKAGE SELECTION	PRICE	
___	8 Hour Course / 1 Review Guide	$120.00	___
___	15 Hour Course / 1 Review Guide	$190.00	___
___	FNP Package	$415.00	___

FNP Package consists of Adult NP, Pediatric NP, Women's Health Care NP Guides & Audio Cassettes of the ANP, PNP, and Childbearing Management Courses.

SUB TOTAL: _____

Maryland Residents add 5% sales tax: _____

CEU Fee ($35 per package, except FNP Package $45): OPTIONAL

TOTAL: (Shipping charge included in package rate) _____

RETURN POLICY

Due to the nature of the material contained in the review books and audio cassettes, returns on books ONLY will be accepted one week post delivery. No returns on audio cassettes except for defective audio cassettes which will be replaced.

MAIL TO: Health Leadership Associates, Inc. P.O. Box 59153 Potomac, MD 20859

OR PHONE: (800) 435-4775; (301) 983-2405

OR FAX: (301) 983-2693

12/98

NOTES

NOTES

NOTES

NOTES

NOTES

NOTES

NOTES

NOTES

NOTES

NOTES

NOTES

NOTES

NOTES

NOTES